Managing diabetes

W0050445

Managing diabetes

Managing diabetes

Editors

Jiten Vora
Royal Liverpool University Hospital
Liverpool, UK

Marc Evans
University Hospital of Llandough
Cardiff, UK

With contributions from

Rupa Ahluwalia
Royal Liverpool and Broadgreen University Hospital

Frank Joseph
Countess of Chester Hospital NHS Foundation Trust

Nagaraj Malipatil
Royal Liverpool and Broadgreen University Hospital

Santosh Shankarnarayan
Royal Liverpool University Hospital

Gayatri Sreemantula
Glan Clwyd Hospital

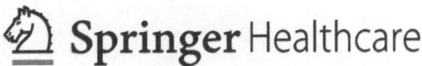

Published by Springer Healthcare Ltd, 236 Gray's Inn Road, London, WC1X 8HB, UK.

www.springerhealthcare.com

© 2012 Springer Healthcare, a part of Springer Science+Business Media.

All rights reserved. No part of this publication may be reproduced, stored in a retrieval system or transmitted in any form or by any means electronic, mechanical, photocopying, recording or otherwise without the prior written permission of the copyright holder.

British Library Cataloguing-in-Publication Data.

A catalogue record for this book is available from the British Library.

ISBN 978-1-908517-57-9

Although every effort has been made to ensure that drug doses and other information are presented accurately in this publication, the ultimate responsibility rests with the prescribing physician. Neither the publisher nor the authors can be held responsible for errors or for any consequences arising from the use of the information contained herein. Any product mentioned in this publication should be used in accordance with the prescribing information prepared by the manufacturers. No claims or endorsements are made for any drug or compound at present under clinical investigation.

Project editors: Hannah Cole and Katrina Dorn
Designer: Joe Harvey
Artworker: Sissan Mollerfors
Production: Marina Maher
Printed in Great Britain by Latimer Trend

Contents

Author biographies

Marc Evans has been a consultant diabetologist at Llandough Hospital and the University Hospital of Wales since the beginning of 2003. He was previously a lecturer in diabetes and endocrinology at the University of Wales College of Medicine. Dr Evans has multiple ongoing academic and clinical interests, including the health economics of diabetes care and health outcomes in people with type 2 diabetes. He has published over 200 articles, book chapters and abstracts and is currently Editor-in-Chief of *Diabetes Therapy*.

Jiten Vora is a consultant physician and honorary professor at the Royal Liverpool University Hospital and the University of Liverpool. He qualified from the University of Cambridge and undertook substantive training in diabetes and endocrinology as a research fellow and then lecturer at the University of Wales College of Medicine. He then undertook a period as a Fulbright senior fellow at Oregon Health Sciences University. He has been a consultant physician and endocrinologist at the Royal Liverpool University Hospital since 1993. He has served on many advisory panels including the National Institute for Clinical Excellence (NICE) and the Diabetes and Renal National Service Frameworks. He has been actively involved in the district-wide delivery of diabetes care.

Professor Vora has ongoing research interests in the development, screening, and treatment of diabetic retinopathy, renal hemodynamics and function, hypertension in type 2 diabetes, renal disease prevention, and the physiological aspects of type 2 diabetes treatment. He has published extensively in these fields.

Rupa Ahluwalia has been a clinical research fellow at the Royal Liverpool & Broadgreen University Hospitals NHS Trust since 2011. She is studying racial differences in the incretin system, which will contribute towards study for an MD at the University of Liverpool. She also holds a Specialist Registrar training number in diabetes and endocrinology in the Mersey Deanery.

Frank Joseph is a consultant physician in endocrinology and diabetes at the Countess of Chester Hospital. He is clinical lead for endocrine services at the Countess of Chester and has a special interest in pituitary disease and metabolic bone disease. He is also clinical lead for diabetes in pregnancy and chair of the North West pre-gestational diabetes audit group. He has an active and diverse research portfolio and publishes on a regular basis.

Dr Joseph is also a member of the Mersey and Cheshire Endocrine Group and is responsible for the nonclinical teaching program for Mersey diabetes and endocrinology trainees and was convener of the first ever Society for Endocrinology Clinical Cases Day in Liverpool, 2011. In addition to his specialty and research interests, he is also Chairman of the New Consultant Committee at the Royal College of Physicians, London and is founder of the Mersey New Consultant Forum.

Nagaraj Malipatil has been a Specialist Registrar in the Mersey Deanery since June 2009. He qualified from Karnataka University Dharwad in India and is currently working and undergoing specialist training in diabetes and endocrinology at the Royal Liverpool University Hospital. Dr Malipatil has special interest in young people with diabetes, obesity, and pituitary disorders.

Santosh Shankarnarayan is enrolled in a medical doctorate program with the University of Liverpool where he is part of a research team studying sclerostin circadian rhythms and its effects on bone mineral metabolism. He is also currently a specialist trainee on the All Wales Diabetes and Endocrinology specialist training program. Dr Shankarnarayan obtained a medical degree in India and has pursued a career in diabetes and endocrinology, including becoming a clinical research fellow at the Royal Liverpool and Broadgreen University Hospitals NHS Trust.

Gayatri Sreemantula graduated with her medical degree in India and attained Higher Specialist training in diabetes, endocrinology, and internal medicine at the Mersey Deanery. Dr Sreemantula currently works as a locum consultant physician at Glan Clwyd Hospital in North Wales.

Chapter 1

Introduction

Frank Joseph and Nagaraj Malipatil

Diabetes is a multisystem disorder characterized by hyperglycemia due to absolute or relative deficiency of insulin, with varying degrees of peripheral resistance to the action of insulin. This condition is predominantly the result of impaired carbohydrate metabolism and, to a lesser extent, impaired protein and lipid metabolism.

Diabetes is associated with reduced life expectancy and is currently the fifth most common cause of death in the world [1]. It is also associated with significant morbidity due to diabetes-related microvascular complications (eg, retinopathy, nephropathy, neuropathy), increased risk of macrovascular complications (eg, ischemic heart disease, stroke, peripheral vascular disease), and diminished health-related quality of life.

The increasing incidence of diabetes has reached epidemic proportions, which has immense implications for the healthcare costs of every nation. It is estimated that if current trends continue, 1 in 8 deaths among 20 to 79 year olds will be attributable to diabetes.

Terminology

Since 1965, the World Health Organization (WHO) has published guidelines for the diagnosis and classification of diabetes. These were last reviewed in 1998 and were published as Guidelines for the Definition, Diagnosis, and Classification of Diabetes Mellitus [2]. Due to accumulating

J. Vora and M. Evans (eds.), *Managing Diabetes*,
DOI: 10.1007/978-1-908517-81-4_1, © Springer Healthcare 2012

data, the American Diabetic Association (ADA) reviewed the diagnostic criteria in 2003 [3]. Currently, the following terminology is in use:

- diabetes mellitus;
- impaired glucose tolerance (IGT);
- impaired fasting glucose (IFG).

Diabetes mellitus

The WHO diagnostic criteria for diabetes are as follows [2]:

- Fasting plasma glucose level ≥7.0 mmol/L (126 mg/dL) or 2 hour plasma glucose ≥11.1 mmol/L (≥200 mg/dL) following ingestion of a 75 g oral glucose load. Fasting is defined as no caloric intake for at least 8 hours.
- In a patient with classic symptoms of hyperglycemia or hyperglycemic crisis, a random plasma glucose ≥11.1 mmol/L (≥200 mg/dL).
- A glycated hemoglobin (HbA1c) level of ≥6.5%.
- In the absence of unequivocal hyperglycemia or symptoms, repeat testing should be carried out 4 to 6 weeks later.

These current diagnostic criteria distinguish a group of individuals with significantly increased premature mortality and increased risk of microvascular as well as cardiovascular complications.

Impaired glucose tolerance

In 1979, the US National Diabetes Data Group (NDDG) [4] recommended the category of IGT to denote a state of increased risk of progressing to diabetes, although it was also noted that many diagnosed with IGT would revert to normal glucose tolerance.

According to the guidelines set by the NDDG, IGT is defined as a fasting glucose <7.0 mmol/L (126 mg/dL) (if measured) and 2 hour glucose ≥7.8 mmol/L (≥140 mg/dL) and <11.1 mmol/L (<200 mg/dL) following a 75 mg oral glucose tolerance test (OGTT). The term IGT was introduced to remove the stigma of diabetes from the term 'prediabetes' (ie, the range between 'normal' and diabetes). IGT is not a clinical entity but is a risk factor for future diabetes and/or adverse outcomes. Studies suggest that IGT is associated with muscle insulin resistance and defective insulin secretion, resulting in less efficient disposal of the glucose load during the OGTT [5].

Impaired fasting glucose

According to the WHO, fasting plasma glucose between ≥6.1 mmol/L and ≤6.9 mmol/L (110 mg/dL and 126 mg/dL) defines IFG. Using these criteria, data from the Diabetes Epidemiology: COllaborative analysis of Diagnostic criteria in Europe (DECODE) study showed that in a European population, 64.8% have isolated IFG, 28.6% have IGT, and 6.6% have diabetes [6]. Similarly, Diabetes Epidemiology: COllaborative analysis of Diagnostic criteria in Asia (DECODA) data showed that in an Asian population, 45.9% have isolated IFG, 35.2% have IGT, and 18.9% have diabetes [7].

The ADA have recommended a lower diagnostic concentration of fasting plasma glucose ≥5.6 mmol/L (100 mg/dL) [3]. People identified using this criterion only have half the risk of developing diabetes and have a more favorable cardiovascular risk profile than those identified using the WHO criteria. There is also a lack of evidence of benefit in terms of progression to diabetes and reducing adverse outcomes at this level (Figure 1.1).

Comparison of World Health Organization (2006) and American Diabetes Association (2003) diagnostic criteria		
Terminology	**WHO 2006**	**ADA 2003**
Diabetes		
Fasting glucose	≥7.0 mmol/L	≥7.0 mmol/L
or	or	or
2 hour glucose*	≥11.1 mmol/L	≥11.1 mmol/L
IGT		
Fasting glucose	<7.0 mmol/L	Not required
2 hour glucose*	≥7.8 and <11.1 mmol/L (if measured)	≥7.8 and <11.1 mmol/L
IFG		
Fasting glucose	≥6.1 and ≤6.9 mmol/L	≥5.6 and ≤6.9mmol/L
2 hour glucose*	Measurement recommended (<7.8 mmol/L if measured)	

Figure 1.1 Comparison of World Health Organization (2006) and American Diabetes Association (2003) diagnostic criteria. *Venous plasma glucose 2 hours after ingestion of 75 g oral glucose load. ADA, American Diabetes Association; IFG, impaired fasting glucose; IGT, impaired glucose tolerance; WHO, World Health Organization.

Etiologic classification of diabetes

The 1997 ADA Expert Committee [8] introduced the terms 'type 1' and 'type 2' diabetes mellitus, and recommended no longer using the terms insulin-dependent, non insulin-dependent, juvenile onset, maturity onset, and adult-onset diabetes.

Type 1 diabetes is characterized by destruction of pancreatic beta cells, leading to absolute insulin deficiency. This is usually due to autoimmune destruction of the pancreatic beta cells (type 1A). Testing postive for islet cell antibodies (ICA) or other autoantibodies (antibodies to glutamic acid decarboxylase [GAD], insulin, and tyrosine phosphatase-like protein [IA-2]) in serum is indicative of immune-mediated or type 1A diabetes. However, some patients have no evidence of autoimmunity and have no other known cause for beta-cell destruction. They are said to have idiopathic diabetes mellitus (type 1B).

Type 2 diabetes is by far the most common type, and is characterized by variable degrees of insulin deficiency and resistance. However, it is occasionally difficult to distinguish between type 1 and atypical presentations of type 2 diabetes. Many patients with type 2 diabetes lose beta-cell function over time and require insulin for glucose control. Thus, the need for insulin does not distinguish between type 1 and type 2 diabetes. Patients with type 2 diabetes typically present with nonketotic hyperglycemia, although ketoacidosis can occur.

In addition to type 1 and type 2 diabetes, specific types of diabetes have been identified: diabetes secondary to diseases of the exocrine pancreas, drugs, or other endocrinopathies (type 3) and gestational diabetes (type 4). This change was an attempt to classify diabetes according to etiologic differences rather than descriptions based upon age at onset or type of treatment (Figure 1.2).

Epidemiology

Every year there are 4 million deaths worldwide due to diabetes [9]. Today, 285 million people across the world are living with diabetes; an estimated 70% are in low and middle income countries [10]. Around 90% of the disease burden is caused by type 2 diabetes, which is a preventable chronic disease [9]. Urbanization, cultural and social factors,

Etiologic classifications of diabetes mellitus

Type 1 diabetes

Immune-mediated

Idiopathic

Type 2 diabetes

Type 3 diabetes

Diseases of the exocrine pancreas

Pancreatitis

Pancreatic trauma/pancreatectomy

Neoplasia

Cystic fibrosis

Hemochromatosis

Endocrinopathies

Acromegaly

Cushing's syndrome

Glucagonoma

Pheochromocytoma

Hyperthyroidism

Somatostatinoma

Conn's syndrome

Drug- or chemical-induced

Thiazides

Glucocorticoids

Diazoxide

Thyroid hormone

Beta-adrenergic agonists

Alpha-interferon

Uncommon forms of immune-mediated diabetes

'Stiff man' syndrome

Anti-insulin receptor antibodies

Syndromes associated with diabetes

Down's syndrome

Klinefelter's syndrome

Turner's syndrome

Huntington's chorea

Freiderich's ataxia

Myotonic dystrophy

Prader-Willi syndrome

Figure 1.2 Etiologic classifications of diabetes mellitus (continues overleaf).

Etiologic classifications of diabetes mellitus (continued)
Type 4 diabetes
Gestational diabetes
Other specific types
Genetic defects of beta cell function
Chromosome 12, HNF-1-alpha (MODY3)
Chromosome 7, glucokinase (MODY2)
Chromosome 20, HNF-4-alpha (MODY1)
Chromosome 13, insulin promoter factor-1 (IPF-1; MODY4)
Chromosome 17, HNF-1-beta (MODY5)
Chromosome 2, NeuroD1 (MODY6)
CEL gene encoding carboxy ester lipase (MODY 7)
Genetic defects in insulin action
Type A insulin resistance
Rabson-Mendenhall syndrome
Lipoatrophic diabetes
Leprechaunism

Figure 1.2 Etiologic classifications of diabetes mellitus (continued). MODY, maturity onset diabetes of the young.

and unhealthy lifestyles are associated with the increase in disease; most of these are modifiable risk factors (Figure 1.3).

There are currently 2.6 million people diagnosed with diabetes in the UK (250,000 of which have type 1), and the number continues to grow [12]. Whilst the risk of developing diabetes increases with age, diabetes is indiscriminate and can affect anyone. However, the burden of the disease tends to fall disproportionately upon people from minority ethnic and lower socioeconomic groups.

The Gonzales group [13] used the UK Health Improvement Network database to estimate the incidence and prevalence of type 1 and type 2 diabetes in the UK general population and found an increase in prevalence from 2.8% in 1996 to 4.3% in 2005 [14]. The incidence of childhood type 1 diabetes varies worldwide, ranging from 0.1 to 37 per 100,000 children under than the age of 15 years [15]. In the UK, the reported incidence is 15 to 17 per 100,000 children. The age of presentation has a bimodal distribution with peaks at 4 to 6 years, and then 10 to 14 years of age [16].

Figures 1.4 and 1.5 summarize key European and global data on diabetes and IGT.

Relative risk for developing type 2 diabetes	
Obesity (BMI, kg/m^2)	**Relative risk**
<23	1.0
23–25	3.0
25–30	8.0
30–35	20.0
>35	40.0
Physical activity (exercise, hours/week)	
>7.0	1.0
4.0–7.0	1.1
2.0–4.0	1.2
0.5–2.0	1.5
<0.5	1.8
Healthy diet (quintiles based on fat/fiber content)	
5	1.00
4	1.15
3	1.30
2	1.50
1	2.00

Figure 1.3 Relative risk for developing type 2 diabetes. A physically inactive individual (<30 min/wk of exercise) who consumes an unhealthy diet (level 1) and is modestly overweight (body mass index [BMI] of 25 to 30) would have a 30-fold (1.8 × 8.0 × 2.0) increased risk of developing type 2 diabetes compared with the general population. This translates to a lifetime risk of nearly 100%. MODY, maturity onset diabetes of the young. Reproduced with permission from Choi and Shi [11].

Risk factors for type 2 diabetes

Diabetes does not impact upon everyone in society equally. Significant inequalities exist in the risk of developing diabetes, as well as in access to health services and the quality of those services. As a result, there are variations in health outcomes, particularly with regard to patients with type 2 diabetes.

Since the early 1990s, the incidence of type 2 diabetes has increased in children and adolescents and is linked to the rise in childhood obesity. Other risk factors are also known to contribute to the development of type 2 diabetes. These include the following:

Ethnicity: Compared with the white UK population, type 2 diabetes is up to six times more common in people of South Asian descent and up to three times more common in those of African and Afro-Caribbean descent. It is also more common in people of Chinese descent and other non-white groups. The average age at diagnosis is also comparatively younger in these groups.

European data on diabetes		
	2010	**2030 (projected)**
Population data		
Total population (millions)	891	897
Adult population (20–79 years, millions)	646	659
Diabetes and IGT in people aged 20–70 years		
Diabetes prevalence (%)	8.5	10.0
IGT prevalence (%)	10.2	11.0
Number of people with diabetes (millions)	55.4	66.5
Number of people with IGT (millions)	66.0	72.2
Number of deaths, male (thousands)	297.6	-
Number of deaths, female (thousands)	336.5	-
Diabetes and IGT in children aged 0–14 years		
Number of children with type 1 diabetes (thousands)	112.0	-
Number of newly diagnosed cases per year (thousands)	17.1	-

Figure 1.4 European data on diabetes. IGT, impaired glucose tolerance.

Global data on diabetes		
	2010	**2030 (projected)**
Population data		
Total population (millions)	7000	8400
Adult population (20–79 years, millions)	4300	5600
Total child population (0–14 years, millions)	1900	
Diabetes and IGT in people aged 20–70 years		
Diabetes prevalence (%)	6.6	7.8
IGT prevalence (%)	7.9	8.4
Number of people with diabetes (millions)	285	438
Number of people with IGT (millions)	344	472
Diabetes and IGT in children aged 0–14 years		
Number of children with type 1 diabetes (thousands)	479.6	
Number of newly diagnosed cases per year (thousands)	75.8	
Annual increase in incidence	3.0	

Figure 1.5 Global data on diabetes. IGT, impaired glucose tolerance.

Advanced age: The prevalence of diabetes rises steeply with age; 1 in 20 people over the age of 65 years in the UK has diabetes and this rises to 1 in 5 people over the age of 85 years [17,18]. The diagnosis of diabetes may be delayed in older people, with symptoms of diabetes often being wrongly attributed to normal aging.

Socioeconomically deprived communities: type 2 diabetes is more prevalent in less affluent populations. Those in the most deprived one-fifth of the population are 2.5 times more likely than average to have diabetes at any given age [19]. Both mortality and morbidity are increased by socioeconomic deprivation. This inequality in outcome has many causes. Whilst deprivation is strongly associated with higher levels of overweight and obesity, physical inactivity, smoking, and poor blood pressure control, other factors include poor blood glucose control, low education levels, lack of employment, low housing status, poor access to services, and referral bias [19].

Gender: Conditions that increase insulin resistance (eg, polycystic ovary syndrome) are also associated with type 2 diabetes. Girls are 1.3 to 1.7 times more likely than boys to develop type 2 diabetes in childhood [20].

Diagnosis

Based on WHO diagnostic criteria, a diagnosis of diabetes mellitus can be made in one of three ways. Unless unequivocal hyperglycemia is present, the diagnosis should be confirmed by repeat testing on a different day.

Diagnosis of type 1 diabetes

Childhood type 1 diabetes usually presents with the classic signs and symptoms resulting from hyperglycemia, including polyuria, polydipsia, weight loss, and lethargy. Diabetic ketoacidosis is often the initial presentation of type 1 diabetes, especially in children younger than 6 years of age, and in children of all ages with poor access to health care. Although there is no diagnostic test, type 1 diabetes is suggested by the presence of serum autoantibodies to islet cells (Figure 1.6), glutamic acid decarboxylase (GAD), the 40K fragment of tyrosine phosphatase (IA-2), and/or decreased insulin production.

Islet cell autoantibodies in type 1 diabetes

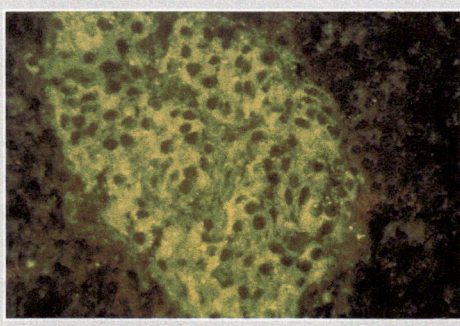

Figure 1.6 Islet cell autoantibodies in type 1 diabetes. Reproduced with permission from Atkinson and Skyler [21].

Diagnosis of type 2 diabetes

Type 2 diabetes is distinguished from other causes of diabetes by clinical presentation and patient history. Although there is no single diagnostic test, type 2 diabetes is suggested by the presence of excess weight, symptoms of insulin resistance (eg, acanthosis nigricans, hypertension, dyslipidemia, polycystic ovary syndrome), a positive family history, and being a member of a high-risk ethnic group.

Glycated hemoglobin for the diagnosis of diabetes

As the measurement of glycated hemoglobin (HbA1c) has become routine in patients with diabetes, it has been the suggested that it could possibly be used as a diagnostic test for diabetes. Two recent reports by an International Expert Committee (comprising members appointed by the ADA, European Association for the Study of Diabetes [EASD], and the International Diabetes Federation [IDF]) have recommended incorporating HbA1c into the current diagnostic criteria [22,23]. The committee recommended that diagnosis of type 2 diabetes should now usually be made solely on the basis of an HbA1c confirmed to be ≥48 mmol/mol (>6.5% HbA1c), without the need to measure a plasma glucose concentration [23]. A 'sub-diabetic high risk state' would exist with an HbA1c measurement of 42–46 mmol/mol (6.0–6.4% HbA1c).

The ADA has ratified the use of both the test and the diagnostic threshold as a fourth way of diagnosing diabetes (as previously discussed, the other three continuing to be a fasting glucose value ≥7 mmol/L, a 2-hour post-OGTT value of ≥11.1 mmol/L or, in someone with classic symptoms of diabetes, a random plasma glucose of ≥11.1 mmol/L) [24]. HbA1c can be used as a diagnostic test for diabetes providing that stringent quality assurance tests are in place, assays are standardized to criteria aligned to the international reference values, and there are no conditions present which preclude its accurate measurement [25].

The following is practical guidance in order to help implement the WHO guidance in the UK [25] (Figure 1.7):

Advantages and disadvantages to using plasma glucose and HbA1c thresholds for the diagnosis of diabetes		
Method	**Advantages**	**Disadvantages**
Fasting and /or post challenge glucose measurements	• Established as the current means of diagnosing diabetes • Directly measures the molecule thought to cause diabetes complications • Not subject to misleading results due to non-glycemic factors • Smaller differences in results between laboratories compared to HbA1c • Less expensive to measure than HbA1c	• Requires patient to be tested in the fasting state and for the sample to be analyzed promptly • May require a glucose tolerance test for diagnosis • A measurement of glucose at a single time-point • Higher within-individual variability than that of HbA1c • Oral glucose tolerance testing is laborious and time consuming
HbA1c	• Established as a means of monitoring patients already known to have diabetes • Does not require a fasting sample and is more stable after sample collection than glucose • A marker of glucose control over the previous weeks/months • Lower within-individual variability than that of glucose • Although more costly than glucose, overall cost as part of a screening/ diagnostic pathway may not be	• Measurement can be misleading in patients with hemoglobinopathies, anemia, or renal failure. • May differ between patients of different ages and ethnicity • Larger differences in results between laboratories compared to glucose • A surrogate marker of hyperglycemia with between-individual discrepancies between glucose and HbA1c

Figure 1.7 Advantages and disadvantages to using plasma glucose and HbA1c thresholds for the diagnosis of diabetes. HbA1c, glycated hemoglobin. Reproduced with permission from Kilpatrick et al [24].

- the finger-prick method of obtaining an HbA1c measurement should not be used unless the methodology used adheres to a national quality assurance scheme that matches the quality assurance results found in laboratories. Finger-prick tests must be confirmed by laboratory-tested venous HbA1c in all patients;
- in patients without symptoms of diabetes, laboratory venous HbA1c tests should be repeated. If the second sample is <48 mmol/mol (<6.5%), the patient should be treated as high-risk for developing diabetes and repeat the test in 6 months (or sooner if symptoms develop).

Situations where solely testing HbA1c is not appropriate for the diagnosis of diabetes [25] (Figure 1.8):

- all children and adolescents;
- patients of any age suspected of having type 1 diabetes;
- patients with symptoms of diabetes lasting less than 2 months;
- patients at high risk of developing diabetes and are acutely ill (eg, those requiring hospital admission);
- patients taking medication that may cause rapid glucose rise (eg, steroids, antipsychotics);
- patients with acute pancreatic damage, including previous pancreatic surgery;

Suggested diabetes screening algorithm

1. Consider laboratory testing of HbA1c as an alternative test in adults without conditions known to affect HbA1c measurement. Do not use if type 1 diabetes is suspected
2. If HbA1c < 40 mmol/mol (<5.8%), diabetes diagnosis is excluded
3. If HbA1c > 55 mmol/mol (>7.2%) on two occasions then diabetes is diagnosed*
4. If HbA1c is 41–54 mmol/mol (5.8–7.2%) [intermediate HbA1c], or an HbA1c >55 mmol/mol (>7.2%) is not confirmed, use existing fasting glucose and/or glucose tolerance test criteria to confirm or exclude diabetes
5. Where HbA1c measurement may be, or is known to be, inappropriate, test patient using existing fasting glucose and/or glucose tolerance test criteria
6. Annual testing is suggested for patients identified as having intermediate HbA1c, IFG, or IGT on initial screening

Figure 1.8 Suggested diabetes screening algorithm. HbA1c, glycated hemoglobin; IFG, impaired fasting glucose; IGT, impaired glucose tolerance. * Repeat testing can be at any time after the initial request and is mainly to ensure a sample mix-up could not have occurred. Adapted with permission from Kilpatrick et al [5].

- in pregnancy;
- presence of genetic, hematologic, and illness-related factors that may influence HbA1c levels.

Differential diagnosis between types of diabetes mellitus

The current classification of diabetes mellitus does not reflect the clinical heterogeneity of patients with diabetes nor the emergence of the concept that early beta-cell dysfunction is likely to be a primary defect in the pathophysiology of diabetes, regardless of 'type.' Other classification schemes have been proposed, accounting for beta-cell autoimmunity, beta-cell function, clinical features, and body weight.

When the diagnosis of type 1 or type 2 diabetes is uncertain by clinical presentation, antibody testing is recommended to differentiate between the two (Figure 1.9) [22]. If there is confirmed autoimmune dysfunction, or there is reason to suspect type 1 diabetes on other clinical grounds, the patient should be presumed to have type 1 diabetes and should be treated with insulin replacement therapy [26]. Given the risk of ketoacidosis, if there is evidence of catabolism (weight loss or dehydration in the setting

Differential diagnosis of diabetes			
	Type 1 diabetes	**Type 2 diabetes**	**Mature-onset diabetes of the young**
Pathogenesis	Beta-cell failure	Beta-cell dysfunction /insulin resistance	Beta-cell dysfunction due to a genetic defect
Body mass index	<24% overweight	85% overweight	Normal/overweight
Family history	5% with family history	75–100% with family history	Autosomal dominant inheritance
Gender	F = M	F > M	F = M
Age of onset	Peak at 10–14 yrs	Peak in middle age	Onset at birth/peak at 2nd–3rd decade of life
Autoimmunity	ICA – positive (70–80%) GAD positive (85–98%)	ICA – negative GAD – may be positive	ICA & GAD – negative
Treatment	Almost always will need insulin eventually	Oral medications 17–37% will need insulin at onset	Diet Life style modification Insulin

Figure 1.9 Differential diagnosis of diabetes. F, female; GAD, glutamic acid decarboxglase; ICA, islet cell antibodies; M, male.

of hyperglycemia) or increased ketogenesis (ketonuria or acidosis), insulin should be started in any patient, regardless of whether they are thought to have type 1 or type 2 diabetes [26].

Screening for diabetes mellitus

Type 2 diabetes can remain hidden and asymptomatic for long periods (often many years), either as pre-diabetic 'metabolic syndrome' or IGT. Diabetes UK estimates that many patients with type 2 diabetes have the condition for 9 to 12 years before diagnosis [12]. Given that many people are not diagnosed with preexisting type 2 diabetes until the time of an acute cardiovascular event, there is debate as to the merit of population-wide screening for diabetes.

The evidence base for diabetic screening

Screening of an older, predominantly white, socially representative cohort of patients enrolled in population-based heart disease studies has revealed a prevalence of undiagnosed frank type 2 diabetes in this group of approximately 7%, while IGT had a prevalence of approximately 20% [27].

There is good evidence that an appropriately designed and targeted screening strategy is effective at detecting undiagnosed type 2 diabetes in a UK-based primary care setting, and that the number of patients needing to be screened to detect one case of type 2 diabetes or IFG is relatively low at 7–13 [28]. Accordingly, the UK Department of Health has announced a series of pilot programs based in inner-city general practitioner surgeries to assess the real-world effectiveness of such screening strategies.

Screening for diabetes appears to be most cost-effective for the 40 to 70-year age band, more so than for the older age bands [29]. Screening is also more cost-effective for people in the hypertensive and obese subgroups, and the costs of screening are offset in many groups by lowering future treatment costs.

The following five criteria define the optimal conditions for screening for diabetes:

- diabetes is an important public health problem;
- an early asymptomatic stage exists;

- there is a suitable screening test available;
- an accepted treatment is available;
- there is evidence that early treatment during the asymptomatic stage improves long-term outcome.

Who should be screened for type 2 diabetes?

There are no agreed hard and fast criteria for selection of the screening population. Screening on the basis of age alone has been shown to have a low yield [27,30]. Most studies have used some or all of the following criteria:

- age >45–50;
- body mass index >27–30 kg/m^2;
- belonging to a high-risk ethnic group for type 2 diabetes (eg, UK-based Afro-Caribbean or Asian-origin populations);
- family history;
- large waist circumference (>35 inches in women and >40 inches in men);
- sedentary lifestyle.

Other criteria might include:

- history of cardiovascular disease;
- history of gestational diabetes;
- obese women with polycystic ovarian syndrome;
- previous evidence of IGT.

Screening tests

The most commonly used screening tests for type 2 diabetes include:

- measurement of fasting plasma glucose (FPG);
- 2-hour plasma glucose during an OGTT.

The results of screening test results should be interpreted as follows [4]:

- fasting or random plasma glucose on one reading of ≥11.1 mmol/L is diagnostic of diabetes;
- two separate results of glucose levels ≥7.0 mmol/L is diagnostic of diabetes;
- if fasting plasma glucose ≥6.1 mmol/L, recall patient for further testing;

- fasting plasma glucose of 6.1–6.9 mmol/L, is defined as IFG and the patient should be screened again after a year;
- fasting plasma glucose of <6.1 mmol/L suggests that the patient is unlikely to have impaired glucose metabolism but should be re-enlisted for further screening at a later date (within 3 years).

References

1 Roglic G, Unwin N, Bennett PH, et al. The burden of mortality attributable to diabetes: realistic estimates for the year 2000. *Diabetes Care.* 2005;28:2130-2135.

2 World Health Organization. Definition, diagnosis and classification of diabetes mellitus and intermediate hyperglycemia. WHO website. www.idf.org/webdata/docs/WHO_IDE_definition_diagnosis_of_diabetes.pdf. Accessed September 5, 2012.

3 Genuth S, Alberti KG, Bennett P, et al. The Expert Committee on the diagnosis and classification of diabetes mellitus. Follow-up report on the diagnosis of diabetes mellitus. *Diabetes Care.* 2003;26:3160-3167.

4 National Diabetes Data Group. Classification and diagnosis of diabetes mellitus and other categories of glucose intolerance. *Diabetes.* 1979;28:1039-1057.

5 Abdul-Ghani MA, Jenkinson CP, Richardson DK, Tripathy D, DeFronzo RA. Insulin secretion and action in subjects with impaired fasting glucose and impaired glucose tolerance. Results from the Veterans Administration Genetic Epidemiology Study. *Diabetes.* 2006;55:1430-1435.

6 DECODE Study Group. Age- and sex-specific prevalence of diabetes and impaired glucose regulation in 13 european cohorts. *Diabetes Care.* 2003; 26:61-69.

7 DECODA Study Group. Age- and sex-specific prevalence of diabetes and impaired glucose regulation in 11 Asian Cohorts. *Diabetes Care.* 2003;26:1770-1780.

8 Gavin JR, Alberti KGMM, Davidson BM, et al. The Expert Committee on the Diagnosis and Classification of Diabetes Mellitus: Report of the expert committee on the diagnosis and classification of diabetes mellitus. *Diabetes Care.* 1997;20:1183-1197.

9 Puska P, Roglic G, Porter D. Facts related to chronic diseases: fact sheet - diabetes. World Health Organization. WHO website. www.who.int/hpr/gs.fs.shtml#::FACTS. Accessed September 5, 2012.

10 International Diabetes Federation (IDF). *IDF Diabetes Atlas, Fifth Edition.* Brussles: IDF; 2009.

11 Choi BC, Shi F. Risk factors for diabetes mellitus by age and sex: results of the National Population Health Survey. *Diabetologia.* 2001;44:1221-1231.

12 Diabetes UK. Introduction to Diabetes. www.diabetes.org.uk. Accessed September 5, 2012.

13 Gonzalez EL, Johansson S, Wallander MA, Rodriguez LA. Trends in the prevalence and incidence of diabetes in the UK: 1996–2005. *J Epidemiol Community Health.* 2009;63:332-336.

14 Masso Gonzales EL, Johansson S, Wallander MA, Garcia Rodriguez LA. Trends in prevalence and incidence of diabetes in the UK: 1996-2005. *J Epidemiol Community Health.* 2009;63:332-336.

15 Karvonen M, Viik-Kajander M, Moltchanova E, Libman I, LaPorte R, Tuomilehto J. Incidence of childhood type 1 diabetes worldwide. Diabetes Mondiale (DiaMond) Project Group. *Diabetes Care.* 2010;23:1516-1526.

16 Felner EI, Klitz W, Ham M, et al. Genetic interaction among three genomic regions creates distinct contributions to early- and late-onset type 1 diabetes mellitus. *Pediatr Diabetes.* 2005;6:213-220.

17 Department of Health. *National service framework for diabetes: standards – supplementary information. Health inequalities in diabetes.* London: Department of Health; 2001.

18 The Information Centre (NHS). Health survey for England 2006. IC website. www.ic.nhs.uk/website/publications/HSE06/pdf. Accessed September 5, 2012.

19 All Party Parliamentary Group for Diabetes and Diabetes UK. *Diabetes and the disadvantaged: reducing health inequalities in the UK*. Diabetes UK website. www.diabetes.org/uk/Documents/Reports/Diabetes-disadvantaged-Nov2006.pdf. Accessed September 5, 2012.

20 Rosenbloom AL, Joe JR, Young RS, Winter WE. Emerging epidemic of type 2 diabetes in youth. *Diabetes Care*. 1999;22:345-354.

21 Atkinson M, Skyler J. *Atlas of Clinical Endocrinology*, Volume 2. London:Springer; 2002.

22 Report of the Expert Committee on the diagnosis and classification of diabetes mellitus. *Diabetes Care*. 1997;20:1183-1197.

23 International Expert Committee Report on the role of the HbA1c assay in the diagnosis of diabetes. Diabetes Care. 2009;32:1327-1334.

24 Kilpatrick ES, Winocour PH. ABCD position statement on haemoglobin A1c for the diagnosis of diabetes. *Pract Diab Int*. 2010;27:1-5.

25 World Health Organization. Use of glycated haemoglobin (HbA1c) in the diagnosis of diabetes mellitus. Abbreviated Report of a WHO Consultation. WHO website. www.who.int/diabetes/publications/report-hba1c_2011.pdf. Accessed September 5, 2012.

26 American Diabetes Association. Standards of medical care in diabetes 2010. *Diabetes Care*. 2010;33 (suppl/1):S11-S61.

27 Thomas MC, Walker MK, Emberson JR, et al. Prevalence of undiagnosed type 2 diabetes and impaired fasting glucose in older British men and women. *Diabet Med*. 2005;22:789-793.

28 Greaves CJ, Stead JW, Hattersley AT, et al. A simple pragmatic system for detecting new cases of type 2 diabetes and impaired fasting glycemia in primary care. *Fam Pract*. 2004;21:57-62.

29 Waugh N, Scotland G, McNamee P, et al. Screening for type 2 diabetes: literature review and economic modelling. *Health Technol Asses*. 2007;11:1-125.

30 Ramachandran A, Snehalatha C, Vijay V, et al. Derivation and validation of diabetes risk score for urban Asian Indians. *Diabetes Res Clin Pract*. 2005;70:63-70.

Chapter 2

Management strategies for diabetes
Rupa Ahluwalia

Diabetes remains one of the biggest health challenges in the developed world, with a current prevalence of approximately 4% of the UK general population. In addition, there is an unprecedented rise in the incidence of type 2 diabetes in recent times [1], along with a much earlier age of onset. At the same time, the advent of newer drugs, especially those involving the incretin axis, makes choosing therapeutics a challenging task.

The overall management of diabetes has certainly come a long way. Compared to the early years of conservative approaches, treatment for diabetes has advanced considerably due to newer drugs and the emerging role of organ transplantation as a potential cure for the disease. Given the changing demographics of the current generation of patients, the concept of a 'standard' treatment strategy no longer holds.

In this chapter, we will discuss the various management strategies for diabetes, including nonpharmacological interventions such as dietary and lifestyle advice. Given the complexity of the disease, along with the choice of multiple treatment options, the majority of the discussion will focus on the management of type 2 diabetes. We have also compared the latest guidance from the American Diabetes Association (ADA), European Association for the Study of Diabetes (EASD), and the National Institute of Clinical Excellence (NICE).

J. Vora and M. Evans (eds.), *Managing Diabetes*,
DOI: 10.1007/978-1-908517-81-4_2, © Springer Healthcare 2012

Glycemic goals of treatment

There is good evidence to support controlling hyperglycemia as a means of reducing long-term complications of diabetes. The most crucial studies providing this evidence are the Diabetes Control and Complications Trial (DCCT) [2] and the Stockholm Diabetes Intervention Study (SDID) [3] in type 1 diabetes, along with the UK Prospective Diabetes Study (UKPDS) [4,5] and Kumamoto Study [6] in type 2 diabetes.

The most recent ADA/EASD guidelines (published in April 2012) [7] recommend a 'general' glycemic goal of <7% glycated hemoglobin (HbA1c), with exceptions for certain individuals. The latest update from NICE, released in May 2009 [8], recommends an HbA1c ≥6.5% as the threshold for initiating or up-titrating therapy in general, while ≥7.5% remains the trigger for triple therapy. However both ADA/EASD and NICE guidance caution against adopting a blanket glycemic 'target' for all patient groups. Factors such as life expectancy and risk of hypoglycemia need to be taken into account for each individual before intensifying treatment.

While there is increasing evidence to support aggressive glycemic control at the point of diagnosis in order to improve metabolic memory and induce a state of 'remission' [9–14], there have been recent conflicting data questioning the safety and overall benefit of tighter glycemic control in terms of reducing cardiovascular events [15–17].

Given the current evidence, it is important to individualize such targets after a careful risk-benefit assessment. Along with glycemic targets, aiming for optimum blood pressure and lipid profile should also remain an integral part of diabetes management and reducing the risk of cardiovascular disease.

Importance of lifestyle issues and patient education

Diabetes is a lifelong condition that is essentially managed by the individual and/or a carer. An individual's lifestyle, especially with regard to physical activity and overall caloric intake, has an enormous impact on the course of diabetes. This is of particular relevance in the long-term management of type 2 diabetes due to the progressive nature of the disease. In addition, lifestyle issues are of greater importance due to the unprecedented rise in incidence of diabetes secondary to increasing adiposity levels. Lifestyle advice given in the form of structured education enables self-management and should be at the heart of diabetes care. According to the National Service Framework (NSF) for diabetes, "people with diabetes need the knowledge, skills and motivation to assess their risks, to understand what they will gain from changing their behavior or lifestyle and to act on that understanding by engaging in appropriate behaviors" [18]. In addition, research has shown that patients who never received diabetes education showed a four-fold increased risk of major complications [19]. A Health Commission survey in 2007 suggested that only 11% of people with type 2 diabetes reported being offered structured education [20].

As change in lifestyle warrants a change in behavior, it is usually much more difficult to implement and, hence, can be perceived as a less effective method of managing diabetes. This is perhaps why physicians use pharmacological intervention at an early stage instead of emphasizing the importance of lifestyle change. Nevertheless, the role of lifestyle modification should not be undermined. Targeting the appropriate patient group with an individualized lifestyle plan devised by an expert should remain an integral part of diabetes management. Such advice may be offered one-to-one or in a group session, depending on local arrangements. In addition, the advice needs to be consistent and delivered by trained heathcare professionals with diabetes-related expertise. In the UK, NICE recommends offering structured education at the time of diagnosis, with annual reinforcement and review [8].

Lifestyle intervention also has a role in diabetes prevention, especially in high-risk groups. Also, those with impaired fasting glucose (IFG; fasting glucose of 6.0–6.9 mmol/L) or impaired glucose tolerance (IGT; fasting glucose of <7.0 mmol/L and 2 hour post-glucose readings between 7.8–11.1 mmol/L) are 5 to 15 times more likely to develop type 2 diabetes [21]. Obesity is the strongest risk factor for type 2 diabetes. The National Health and Nutrition Examination Survey III (1998–1994) data showed that the risk of diabetes is approximately 50% in patients with body mass index (BMI) of 30 kg/m^2 or more [22]. Targeted lifestyle intervention can delay or even prevent the incidence of type 2 diabetes in such individuals [23,24].

It is important that we continue to recognise lifestyle modification as a crucial part of preventing and managing diabetes, warranting active participation of both patients and health professionals.

What determines treatment choice?

Broadly speaking, the initial choice of treatment is guided by the type of diabetes. All individuals with suspected or proven type 1 diabetes should be commenced on insulin as first-line treatment.

In type 2 diabetes, treatment is not as straightforward. The initial treatment is guided by the HbA1c at diagnosis, the presence of osmotic symptoms, evidence of catabolic state (rapid unintentional weight loss), and the presence of any organ dysfunction that may preclude the use of a particular therapeutic agent. In addition, other attributes including age, body weight, convenience of administration, and impact on work-related issues (such as driving motor vehicles) also play a crucial role in determining the order of medications used. The efficacy and side effect profile of each drug in the individual patient is also taken into account.

In individuals with an initial HbA1c of <10% in the absence of osmotic symptoms, the general consensus is to start metformin, especially in those who are overweight. Despite an increasing number of options for addressing hypergycemia, only metformin has been shown to improve prognosis as a primary endpoint in a randomized-controlled trial [25]. Sulfonylureas are an option in cases where metformin use is contraindicated or not tolerated. Sulfonylureas are also prescribed where rapid therapeutic response is desired, especially in the symptomatic group.

Initial treatment should be up-titrated at a rapid pace to aim for an agreed target HbA1c. Patients should be made aware of the progressive nature of the disease; after a successful initial response to oral therapy, patients fail to maintain target HbA1c levels (<7%) at a rate of 5–10% per year. An analysis from the UKPDS study found that 50% of patients originally controlled with a single drug required the addition of a second drug after 3 years; after 9 years, 75% of patients needed multiple therapies to achieve the target HbA1c value [26].

Several agents can be considered as add-on therapy when metformin monotherapy fails, including sulfonylureas, thiazolidinediones (TZDs), and alpha-glucosidase inhibitors. Oral agents as monotherapy (TZDs, metformin, repaglinide, alpha-glucosidase inhibitors and sulfonylureas) improve glycemic control to almost the same degree (eg, decrease in HbA1c of approximately 1%) [27]. When combining two antidiabetes drugs, a further 1% HbA1c reduction can be obtained. These agents are discussed in more detail in Chapter 4.

Individuals with markedly raised HbA1c at diagnosis (>10%), with or without osmotic and catabolic symptoms, should be treated more aggressively, with early use of insulin to be considered. This issue is discussed further in Chapter 3.

Current guidelines for treatment

The emergence of new incretin-based drugs makes prescribing in diabetes more exciting but far from easy. Unfamiliarity with these new drugs and relatively higher prescription costs warrants judicious use at this stage.

Clinical guidelines help with this conundrum by bringing the best available evidence to the point of practice. However, guidelines often do not provide recommendations for all clinical scenarios. In this chapter we endeavor to cover the most up-to-date recommendations based on the clinical guidelines from the ADA, EASD, and NICE on the management of type 2 diabetes. By comparing available guidelines, we aim to provide a balanced viewpoint to aid appropriate and effective prescribing for clinicians.

ADA/EASD consensus statement

The latest ADA/EASD consensus statement is based on clinical trial evidence and the clinical judgement of ten named authors [7]. The general glycemic goal advised by the ADA/EASD consensus is a HbA1c level <7%, with recommendations for individualized targets in some patients.

The choice of treatment is based on effectiveness of individual therapies and basal level of glycemic control. In cases of high basal HbA1c (eg, HbA1c >9%), a more aggressive approach using insulin alone or combination therapy is recommended. While metformin remains the 'gold standard' first-line agent, the ADA/EASD guidelines now recommend insulin for many patients at all stages of the disease, including first-line (in the setting of marked uncontrolled hypoglycemia), and/or HbA1c >12%, or the presence of ketonuria or catabolic symptom) [7].

Thiazolidinediones

The ADA/EASD authors advise caution in using TZDs due to increased risks of fluid retention, heart failure, and incidence of fractures [7]. Currently in the US, TZDs are approved for use in combination with metformin, sulfonylureas, glinides, and insulin [28]. The FDA has substantially restricted the use of rosiglitazone by requiring a risk evaluation and mitigation strategy (REMS) due to an increased risk for cardiovascular ischemia [29].

Glucagon-like peptide-1 agonists

The glucagon-like peptide [GLP-1] agonists exenatide and liraglutide are approved for use in the US with sulfonylurea, metformin, and/or a TZD [28]. However, unlike the NICE guidance, the ADA/EASD does not suggest a restriction in use of GLP-1 agonists in individuals with a BMI >35 kg/m^2 [7].

Dipeptidyl peptidase-4 inhibitors

The ADA/EASD authors note that dipeptidyl peptidase-4 (DPP-4) inhibitors have 'intermediate' efficacy in combination with metformin. They can also be used in a triple combination with metformin plus a sulfonylurea, TZD, or insulin. These inhibitors are weight-neutral and have been found to be well tolerated [7].

Insulin

The updated ADA/EASD guidelines recommend starting most patients with basil insulin. Rapid insulin analog preparations should be used for patients who need prandial insulin therapy due to diminished insulin secretory capacity [7].

Initiating therapy

The ADA/EASD's general recommendations are found in Figure 2.1. All patients should start by making lifestyle changes, such as healthy eating and increased exercise, and continue with these changes for the duration.

ADA/EASD general recommendations for antiglycemic therapy in type 2 diabetes

Healthy eating, weight control, increased physical activity

Initial drug monotherapy	Metformin
Efficacy (↓ HbA1C)	High
Hypoglycemia	Low risk
Weight	Neutral/loss
Side effects	GI/lactic acidosis

If needed to reach individualized HbA1C target after ~3 months, proceed to two-drug combination (order not meant to denote any specific preference):

Two-drug combinations*	Metformin + Sulfonylurea**	Metformin + TZD	Metformin + DPP-4 inhibitor	Metformin + GLP-1 receptor agonist	Metformin + Insulin (usually basal)
Efficacy (↓ HbA1C)	High	High	Intermediate	High	Highest
Hypoglycemia	Moderate risk	Low risk	Low risk	Low risk	High risk
Weight	Gain	Gain	Neutral	Loss	Gain
Major side effect(s)	Hypoglycemia	Edema, HF, Fx's	Rare	GI	Hypoglycemia

If needed to reach individualized HbA1C target after ~3 months, proceed to two-drug combination (order not meant to denote any specific preference):

Three-drug combinations	Metformin + Sulfonylurea† + TZD or DPP-4-i or GLP-1-RA or insulin‡	Metformin + TZD + SU† or DPP-4-i or GLP-1-RA or insulin‡	Metformin + DPP-4 inhibitor + SU† or TZD or insulin‡	Metformin + GLP-1 receptor agonist + SU† or TZD or insulin‡	Metformin + Insulin (usually basal) + TZD or DPP-4-i or GLP-1-RA

If combination therapy that includes basal insulin has failed to achieve HbA1C target after 3–6 months, proceed to a more complex insulin strategy, usually in combination with one or two non-insulin agents:

More complex insulin strategies	Insulin (multiple daily doses)

Figure 2.1 ADA/EASD general recommendations for antiglycemic therapy in type 2 diabetes. Reinforce lifestyle interventions at every visit and check HbA1c every 3 months until <7%, and then every 6 months. The interventions should be changed if HbA1c is ≥7%. ADA, American Diabetes Association; EASD, European Association for the Study of Diabetes; DPP-4, dipeptidyl peptidase-4; Fx, fracture; GLP-1-RA, glucagon-like peptide-1 receptor agonists; HbA1c, glycated hemoglobin; HF, heart failure; GI, gastrointestinal; SU, sulfonylurea; TZD, thiazolidinedione. *Consider beginning at this stage in patients with very high HbA1c (eg. <9%). **Consider rapid-acting, non-sulfonylurea secretagogues (meglitinides) in patients with irregular meal schedules or who develop late postprandial hypoglycemia on sulfonylureas. ‡Usually a basal insulin (NPH, glargine, detemir) in combination with noninsulin agents. Adapted with permission from Inzucchi et al 2012 [7].

Metformin therapy can be started at diagnosis or soon afterwards. If the target HbA1c is not reached after about 3 months, a sulfonyurea, a TZD, GLP-1 receptor antagonist, DPP-4 inhibitor, or basal insulin can be added to metformin. Three-drug combinations may also be considered. If the patient is taking insulin as part of a combination therapy regimen and their HbA1c levels have not lowered to target after 3–6 months, a more complex insulin strategy will need to be tried [7].

NICE recommendations

The latest NICE guidance (issued in May 2009) continues to recommend an HbA1c ≥6.5% as the threshold for initiating or up titrating therapy, while HbA1c ≥7.5% remains the trigger for triple therapy (Figure 2.2) [8].

NICE continues to recommend metformin as first-line treatment and sulfonylureas as second-line agents.

DPP-4 inhibitors

Compared to the ADA/EASD, NICE does offer more clarity in terms of role for DPP-4 inhibitors (eg, sitagliptin, vildagliptin) in the treatment algorithm. They are recommended instead of a sulfonylurea or metformin as second-line agents in those who are unable to take the combination due to intolerance or contraindication of use of either of the drugs. The guidelines emphasize the need to avoid sulfonylurea use in patients with increased risk of hypoglycemia.

Sitagliptin, the only DPP-4 inhibitor available at the time of publication of the NICE guideline, is also recommended as a third-line agent in combination with metformin and a sulfonylurea when insulin is unacceptable or inappropriate.

Thiazolidinediones

NICE recommends considering a TZD (eg, piogitazone) as a second-line agent with either metformin or a sulfonylurea, similar to a DPP-4 inhibitors, or as third-line therapy in combination with metformin and a sulfonylurea with suboptimal control, where insulin is inappropriate [8]. NICE clearly recommends not continuing or commencing a TZD in people who have heart failure, or who are at higher risk of fracture [8].

The combination of insulin and pioglitazone continues to be recommended as an option in selected patients. The NICE guidelines suggest that TZD may be preferable to a DPP-4 inhibitor in case of marked insulin insensitivity, or if a DPP-4 inhibitor is contraindicated, or not preferred due to previous intolerance or poor response.

DPP-4 inhibitor and TZD should be continued only if there is evidence of a beneficial metabolic response (eg, a reduction of at least 0.5% HbA1c in 6 months).

Due to ongoing concerns of increased risk of cardiovascular disease associated with the use of rosiglitazone, the European Medicines Agency Committee for Medicinal Products for Humane Use (EMA CHMP) recommended the suspension of marketing of rosigltazone across the UK from September 2010 [30].

GLP-1 mimetic

GLP-1 mimetic (exenatide) use is limited as a third-line treatment in individuals with a BMI ≥35 kg/m^2 in those of European descent (with appropriate adjustment for other ethnic groups), or a BMI <35 kg/m^2 in patients for whom insulin therapy would have significant occupational implications or weight loss would benefit other significant obesity-related comorbidities. NICE recommends continuing GLP-1 mimetic therapy only if there is evidence of a beneficial metabolic response (eg, a HbA1c reduction of at least 1.0% and a weight loss of at least 3% of initial body weight after 6 months).

Long-acting human insulin analogs

Similar to the ADA/EASD guidance, NICE recommends insulin as a step-up option after triple therapy, or after dual therapy in case of suboptimal glycemic control.

A long-acting insulin analog (eg, insulin detemir, insulin glargine) is recommended over neutral protamine hagedorn insulin in people with significant hypoglycemia, device preference, or those who want to reduce the number of injections. Similarly, premixed preparations with short-acting insulin analogs are indicated when there is preference for injecting insulin immediately before a meal, or due to hypoglycemia or marked post-prandial hyperglycemia.

NICE guideline on type 2 diabetes

Blood glucose-lowering therapy

HbA1c ≥6.5%* after trial of lifestyle interventions

↓

Metformin†

↓

| HbA1c ≥6.5%* | HbA1c <6.5%* Monitor for deterioration |

↓

Metformin + sulfonylurea§

↓

| HbA1c ≥7.5%* | HbA1c <7.5%* Monitor for deterioration |

↓

Add insulin†,‡, particularly if the person is markedly hyperglycemic

Insulin + metformin + sulfonylurea§

↓

| HbA1c ≥7.5%* | HbA1c <7.5%* Monitor for deterioration |

Consider sulfonylurea§ here if:
- patient is not overweight (tailor the assessment of body weight-associated risk according to ethnic group‡), or
- metformin is not tolerated or is contraindicated, or
- a rapid therapeutic response is required because of hyperglycemic symptoms

Consider a rapid-acting insulin secretagogue for people with erratic lifestyles

Consider substituting a DPP-4 inhibitor§§ or a thiazolidinedione¶¶ for the sulfonylurea if there is a significant risk of hypoglycemia (or its consequences) or a sulfonylurea is contraindicated or not tolerated

Consider adding sitagliptin or a thiazolidinedione¶¶ instead of insulin if insulin is unacceptable (because of employment, social, recreational or other personal issues, or obesity)

Consider adding exenatide** to metformin and a sulfonylurea if:
- BMI ≥35 kg/m² in people of European descent†† and there are problems associated with high weight, or
- BMI <35 kg/m² and insulin is unacceptable because of occupational implications or weight loss would benefit other comorbidities

Increase insulin dose and intensify regimen over time

Consider pioglitazone with insulin if:
- a thiazolidinedione has previously had a marked glucose-lowering iffect, or
- blood glucose control is inadequate with high-dose insulin

Figure 2.2 NICE guideline on type 2 diabetes. *Or individually agreed target. †With active dose titration. ‡See the NICE clinical guideline on obesity (www.nice.org.uk/CG43). §Offer once-daily sulfonylurea if adherence is a problem. ¶Only continue DPP-4 inhibitor or thiazolidinedione if reduction in HbA1c of at least 0.5% points in 6 months. **Only continue exenatide if reduction in HbA1c of at least 1% point and weight loss of at least 3% of initial body weight at 6 months.

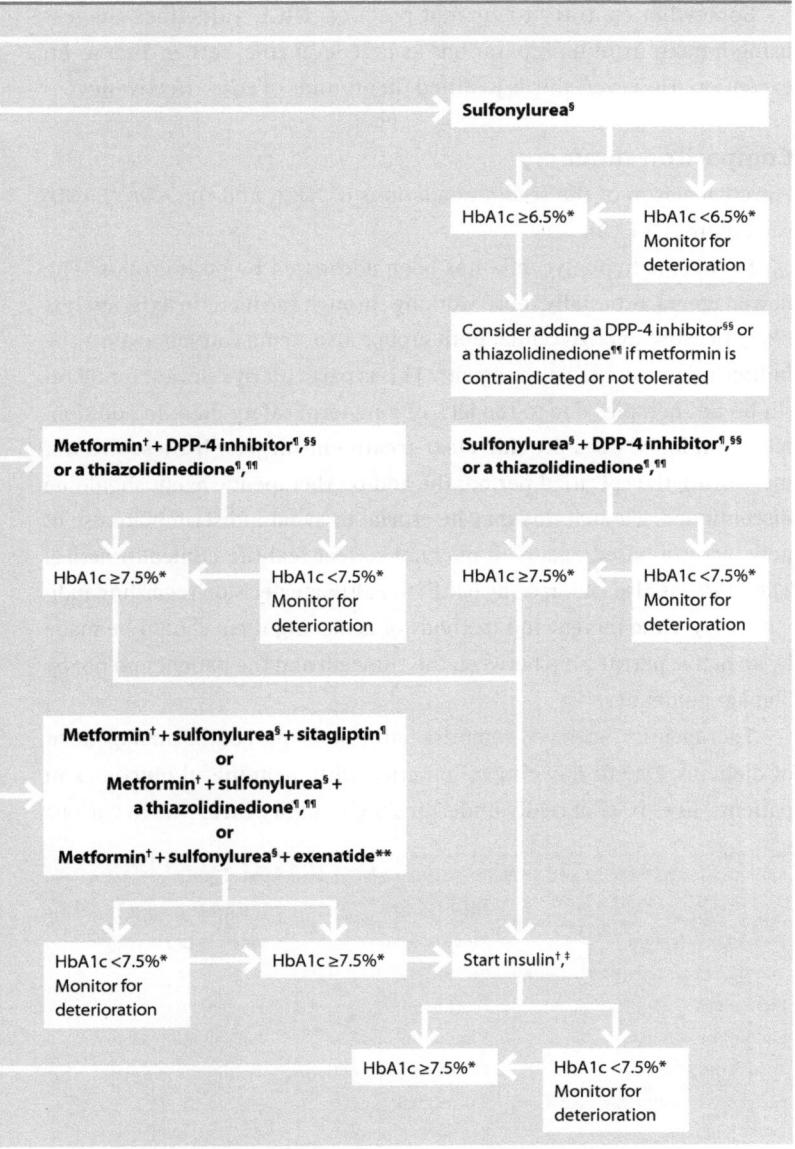

Sulfonylurea§

HbA1c ≥6.5%* → HbA1c <6.5%*
Monitor for
deterioration

Consider adding a DPP-4 inhibitor§§ or
a thiazolidinedione¶¶ if metformin is
contraindicated or not tolerated

Metformin† + DPP-4 inhibitor¶,§§
or a thiazolidinedione¶,¶¶

Sulfonylurea§ + DPP-4 inhibitor¶,§§
or a thiazolidinedione¶,¶¶

HbA1c ≥7.5%* ← HbA1c <7.5%*
Monitor for
deterioration

HbA1c ≥7.5%* ← HbA1c <7.5%*
Monitor for
deterioration

Metformin† + sulfonylurea§ + sitagliptin¶
or
Metformin† + sulfonylurea§ +
a thiazolidinedione¶,¶¶
or
Metformin† + sulfonylurea§ + exenatide**

HbA1c <7.5%* → HbA1c ≥7.5%* → Start insulin†,‡
Monitor for
deterioration

HbA1c ≥7.5%* ← HbA1c <7.5%*
Monitor for
deterioration

††With adjustment for other ethnic groups. ‡‡Continue with metformin and sulfonylurea (and acarbose, if used), but only continue other drugs that are licensed for use with insulin. Review the use of sulfonylurea if hypoglycemia occurs. §§DPP-4 inhibitor refers to sitagliptin or vildagliptin. ¶¶Thiazolidinedione refers to pioglitazone. NICE, National Institute for Health and Clinical Excellence. Reproduced with permission from NICE 2009 [8].

Somewhat contrary to current practice, NICE guidelines suggest using human insulin preparations as a general rule, rather than as an exception. However, this is justified on grounds of cost-effectiveness.

Comparison summary

For comparison of the recommendations of NICE and the ADA/EASD, see Figure 2.3 [7,8].

Iatrogenic hypoglycemia has been addressed by both groups. The newer agents, especially those working through the incretin axis, are less likely to cause hypoglycemia. Both groups also sound caution against the indiscriminate use of newer agents. This is particularly relevant for incretin-based therapies due to the lack of long-term safety data. In addition, NICE guidance does provide clear treatment targets: if these are not met during the specified period, the add-on therapeutic agent should be discontinued. Though this may be crucial to avoid indiscriminate use of new incretin-based agents, it may not reflect real-life clinical practice. Therefore, as also endorsed by NICE, the ultimate decision regarding individual glycemic targets and methods of achieving them should be made by an active partnership between the clinician and the patient and not by blanket guidelines.

Therapeutics, however, comprise only a small part of the management of diabetes. Day-to-day clinical practice with meaningful outcomes in patients' lives is what really underpins high-quality care. Due to various

Comparisons of the recommendations of NICE and ADA/EASD		
	NICE	ADA/EASD
Date of publication	May 2009	April 2012
Threshold for action (HbA1c values)	>6.5%	>7%
Metformin	First line	First line
Sulfonylureas	First line/second line	Second line/third line
Thiazolidinediones	Pioglitazone/rosiglitazone	Pioglitazone
GLP-1 receptor agonists	BMI restriction	–
DPP-4 inhibitors	Second line/third line	Second line/third line

Figure 2.3 Comparisons of the recommendations of NICE and ADA/EASD. ADA, American Diabetes Association; BMI, body mass index; DPP-4 inhibitors, dipeptidyl peptidase-4 inhibitors; EASD; European Association for the Study of Diabetes; HbA1c; glycated hemoglobin; NICE, National Institute of Clinical Excellence.

factors, including treatment inertia, there are wide gaps between recommendations and clinical practice. Also, with the current move towards a 'pay for performance' culture in health care and a focus on predetermined 'outcome' targets [31], patient-centered care appears to be under threat. This is likely to be detrimental for patients with chronic disease such as diabetes where care plans have to be individually tailored.

While the ADA/EASD consensus group may allow flexibility in treatment strategy by suggesting a two-tier approach, NICE guidance is based on up-to-date evidence and aids in translating recommendations into real-world clinical practice. It also helps the individual physician to tailor treatment based on patients' needs, rather than purely upon predetermined outcome targets.

References

1   Shaw JE, Sicree RA, Zimmet PZ. Global estimates of the prevalence of diabetes for 2010 and 2030. *Diabetes Res Clin Pract*. 2009;87:4-14.

2   Diabetes Control and Complications Trial Research Group. The effect of intensive diabetes treatment on the development and progression of long-term complications in insulin-dependent diabetes mellitus: the Diabetes Control and Complications Trial. *N Engl J Med*. 1993;329:978-986.

3   Reichard P, Nilsson B-Y, Rosenqvist U. The effect of long-term intensified insulin treatment on the development of microvascular complications of diabetes mellitus. *N Engl J Med*. 1993;329:304-309.

4   UK Prospective Diabetes Study (UKPDS) Group. Intensive blood glucose control with sulphonylureas or insulin compared with conventional treatment and risk of complication in patients with type 2 diabetes (UKPDS 33). *Lancet*. 1998;352:837-853.

5   UK Prospective Diabetes Study (UKPDS) Group. Effect of intensive blood glucose control with metformin on complication in overweight patients with type 2 diabetes (UKPDS 34). *Lancet*. 1998;352:854-865.

6   Ohkubo Y, Kishikawa H, Araki E, et al. Intensive insulin therapy prevents the progression of diabetic microvascular complications in Japanese patients with NIDDM: a randomised prospective 6-year study. *Diabetes Res Clin Pract*. 1995;28:103-117.

7   Inzucchi SE, Bergenstal RM, Buse JB, et al. Management of hyperglycaemia in type 2 diabetes: a patient-centered approach. Position statement of the American Diabetes Association (ADA) and the European Association for the Study of Diabetes (EASD). *Diabetologia*. 2012;55:1577-1596.

8   National Institute for Health and Clinical Excellence. Type 2 diabetes: newer agents for blood glucose control in type 2 diabetes (Clinical guideline 87). 2009. www.nice.org.uk/CG87. Accessed September 5, 2012.

9   Weng JP, Li YB, Xu W, et al. Effect of intensive insulin therapy on β-cell function and glycaemic control in patients with newly diagnosed type 2 diabetes: a multicentre randomised parallel-group trial. *Lancet*. 2008;371:1753-1760.

10 Ilkova H, Glaser B, Tunckale A, Bagriacik N, Cerasi E. Induction of long-term glycemic control in newly diagnosed type 2 diabetic patients by transient intensive insulin treatment. *Diabetes Care*. 1997;20:1353-1356.

11 Weng JP, Li YB, Xu W, et al. The effect of short-term continuous subcutaneous insulin infusion treatment on beta-cell function in newly diagnosed type 2 diabetic patients. *Chin J Diabetes (Chin)*. 2003;11:10-15.

12 Zhu F, Ji LN, Han XY, et al. Induction of long-term glycemic control in newly diagnosed type 2 diabetic patients by transient intensive insulin treatment. *Chin J Diabetes (Chin)*. 2003;11:5-9.

13 Ryan EA, Imes S, Wallace C. Short-term intensive insulin therapy in newly diagnosed type 2 diabetes. *Diabetes Care*. 2004;27:1028-1032.

14 Li YB, Xu W, Liao ZH, et al. Induction of long-term glycemic control in newly diagnosed type 2 diabetic patients is associated with improvement of β-cell function. *Diabetes Care*. 2004; 27:2597-2602.

15 ADVANCE Collaborative Group. Intensive blood glucose control and vascular outcomes in patients with type 2 diabetes. *N Engl J Med*. 2008;358:260-272.

16 Duckworth W, Abraira C, Mortiz T, et al; for the VADT Investigators. Glucose control and vascular complications in veterans with type 2 diabetes. *N Engl J Med*. 2009;360:129-139.

17 Action to Control Cardiovascular Risk in Diabetes Study Group. Effects of intensive glucose lowering in type 2 diabetes. *N Engl J Med*. 2008;358:2545-2559.

18 Department of Health. National Service Framework for Diabetes: Delivery Strategy; 2003.

19 Nicolucci A, Cavaliere D, Scorpiglione N, et al, A comprehensive assessment of the avoidability of long-term complications of diabetes, *Diabetes Care*. 1996;19:927-933.

20 Healthcare Commission. Managing diabetes: improving services for people with diabetes. www.cqc.org.uk/publications.cfm?fde_id=559. Accessed September 5, 2012.

21 Santaguida PL, Balion C, Hunt D, et al. Diagnosis, prognosis, and treatment of impaired glucose tolerance and impaired fasting glucose. Summary, Evidence Report/Technology Assessment No. 128; 2005. www.ahrq.gov/downloads/pub/evidence/pdf/impglucose/impglucose.pdf. Accessed September 5, 2012.

22 US Department of Health and Human Services. National Center for Health Statistics. Third National Health and Nutrition Examination Survey, 1988-1994 (CD-ROM). Public Use Data File Documentation Number 76200. Hyattsville, MD: Centers for Disease Control and Prevention;1996.

23 Tuomilehto J, Lindstrom J, Eriksson JG, et al. Prevention of type 2 diabetes mellitus by changes in lifestyle among subjects with impaired glucose tolerance. *N Engl J Med*. 2001;344:1343-1350.

24 The Diabetes Prevention Program. Design and methods for a clinical trial in the prevention in type 2 diabetes. *Diabetes Care*. 1999;22:623-634.

25 UK Prospective Diabetes Study (UKPDS) Group. Effect of intensive blood-glucose control with metformin on complications in overweight patients with type 2 diabetes (UKPDS 34). *Lancet*. 1998;352:854-865.

26 Turner RC, Cull CA, Frighi V, Holman RR; for the UK Prospective Diabetes Study (UKPDS) Group. Glycemic control with diet, sulfonylurea, metformin, or insulin in patients with type 2 diabetes mellitus: progressive requirement for multiple therapies. *JAMA*. 1999;281:2005-2012.

27 Bolen S, Wilson L, Vassy J, et al. Comparative effectiveness and safety of oral diabetes medications for adults with type 2 diabetes. Comparative effectiveness review No. 8. Rockville, MD: Agency for Healthcare Research and Quality; 2007. www.effectivehealthcare.ahrq.gov/repFiles/OralFullReport.pdf. Accessed September 5, 2012.

28 Nathan DM, Buse JB, Davidson MB, et al. Medical management of hyperglycemia in type 2 diabetes: a consensus algorithm for the initiation and adjustment of therapy. A consensus Statement of the America Diabetes Association and the European Association for the Study of Diabetes. *Diabetes Care*. 2009;32:193-203.

29 US Food and Drug Administration. "FDA Drug Safety Communication: Avandia (rosiglitazone) labels now contain updated information about cardiovascular risks and use in certain patients." FDA website. www.fda.gov/Drugs/DrugSafety/ucm241411.htm. Accessed September 5, 2012.

30 Medicines and Healthcare products Regulatory Agency. "Europe-wide suspension of marketing authorisation for Avandia, Avandamet and Avaglim (rosiglitazone)." MHRA website. www.mhra.gov.uk/NewsCentre/Pressreleases/CON094127. Accessed September 5, 2012.

31 Department of Health. Annex A: Quality indicators - Summary of points. DHA website. www.dh.gov.uk/prod_consum_dh/groups/dh_digitalassets/documents/digitalasset/dh_120152.pdf. Accessed September 5, 2012.

Chapter 3

Insulin therapies

Gayatri Sreemantula

The discovery of insulin by Banting and Best in 1921 is generally regarded as the greatest advance in modern diabetes management, as insulin can be life saving in type 1 diabetes and health-preserving in type 2 diabetes. Since 1921, remarkable advances in purification techniques, coupled with greater understanding of the nature of physiologic insulin and novel insulin delivery systems, has led to the better diabetes management. From animal insulins to human insulin formulations, followed by analog insulins and inhaled insulins, the evolutionary process continues. In fact, insulin was in use before oral agents, which were only introduced in the mid-1950s.

Mode of action

Insulin binds to insulin receptors throughout the body (Figure 3.1) and promotes the cellular uptake of glucose into fat tissue and skeletal muscle. It also inhibits hepatic glucose output, thus lowering blood glucose levels.

Types of insulin preparations

Currently in the UK, most insulins used are either human or analogs of human insulin. There are at least 11 different insulin preparations available and they can be divided into rapid-, short-, intermediate-, and long-acting, based on their pharmacokinetic properties.

J. Vora and M. Evans (eds.), *Managing Diabetes*,
DOI: 10.1007/978-1-908517-81-4_3, © Springer Healthcare 2012

Structure and function of the insulin receptor

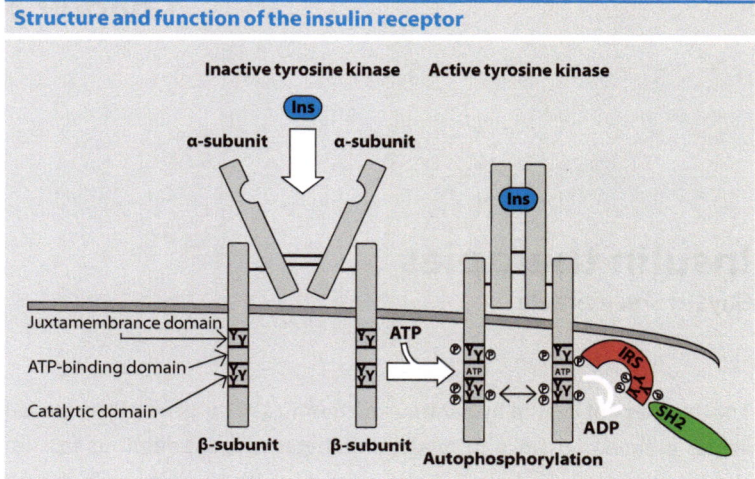

Figure 3.1 Structure and function of the insulin receptor. The binding of insulin to the α subunit of the insulin receptor concentrates insulin at its site of action and induces conformational changes in the receptor. This stimulates tyrosine kinase activity which is intrinsic to the B subunit of the insulin receptor. ADP, adenosine diphosphate; ATP, adenosine triphosphate; Ins, insulin; IRS, insulin receptor substrates; SH2, SRC homolog 2. Adapted from Andreas 2009 [1].

Rapid-acting analog insulins

An analog insulin is a type of insulin that has been structurally modified to improve its pharmokinetic and pharmodynamic properties (compared with regular human insulin), whilst preserving its biological effects and safety profile. They are produced by recombinant DNA techniques that use nonpathogenic laboratory strains of *Escherichia coli*. Three rapid-acting analog insulins are currently in use in the UK: insulin lispro, insulin aspart, and insulin glulisine. All three have an onset of action within 5 to 15 minutes and are used to reduce the peak of glycemia that occurs after meal ingestion. They also have a shorter duration of action when compared with the human soluble insulin. The structures of insulin lispro and insulin aspart are shown in Figure 3.2.

Regular or short-acting insulin

Regular insulin contains zinc-insulin crystals dissolved in a clear fluid in a hexameric form, which dissociates into the active dimeric and monomeric form after a subcutaneous injection, causing a relative delay in the onset

Structures of analog insulins

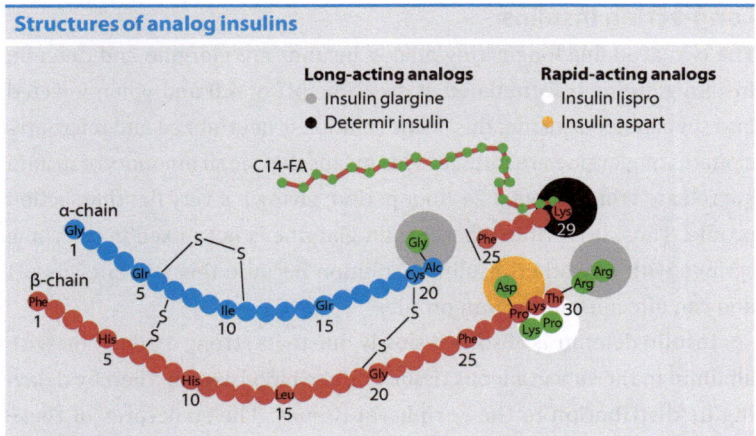

Figure 3.2 Structures of analog insulins. Reproduced with permission from Owens 2002 [2].

and duration of action. Regular insulins are also called clear, neutral, or unmodified insulins. They were the short-acting component of the premixed insulins in the pre-analog era.

Actrapid and Humulin S are commonly used regular insulins. Regular insulins are soluble and are ideally injected 30 to 45 minutes before a meal. Their peak activity occurs after approximately 30 minutes and lasts for about 2 hours (depending on the dose). However, when injected intravenously, the plasma half-life of regular insulin is approximately five minutes, and therefore an infusion is needed for a sustained therapeutic effect. Intravenous insulin infusion is generally used in a hospital setting for rapid normalization of glucose or in emergencies (eg, diabetic ketoacidosis, hyperosmolar hyperglycemic states). Only regular insulins are given intravenously.

Intermediate-acting insulins

Humulin I and Insulatard are intermediate-acting insulins and contain protamine, which prolongs their duration of action when given subcutaneously. Also called neutral protamine hagedorn (NPH), this type of insulin has an onset of action of approximately 2 hours, peak effect at 6 to 14 hours, and duration of action up to 24 hours (depending on the size of the dose). NPH insulin is available in various combinations with either regular insulin or short-acting insulins.

Long-acting insulins

The two available long-acting analog insulins are glargine and detemir. Insulin glargine is formulated at an acidic pH of 4.0 and when injected into subcutaneous tissue, this acidic solution is neutralized and micropre-cipitates of glargine are formed. This means that small amounts of insulin are released throughout a 24-hour period, giving it a very flat time-action profile. Thus, it is critical that insulin glargine is not mixed in the same syringe with any other insulin or solution because this will alter its pH and can affect its absorption profile.

Insulin detemir is absorbed slowly due to its strong association with albumin in the subcutaneous tissue and the bloodstream, thereby delaying its distribution to the peripheral tissues. The structures of these long-acting insulin analogs are shown in Figure 3.2.

Insulin premixes

Insulin premixes are a mixture of short-acting or rapid-acting insulins with an intermediate-acting insulin in a fixed ratio that is suitable for a twice-daily dosage regime. In the pre-analog era, NPH insulin was used in combination with regular insulin (eg, Humulin M3, Insuman Comb 25, Mixtard 30). Now, the premixes are largely biphasic analog insulins (eg, Humalog Mix 25, Novomix 30, Humalog Mix 50).

The shorter-acting component of the insulin premix covers the time between breakfast and lunch, whereas the intermediate-acting NPH insulin peaks around noon and covers the interval from afternoon until dinnertime. The second 'split-mixed' dose is administered before the evening meal and provides insulin coverage during the interval between dinner and bedtime (short-acting insulin component) and lasts overnight (intermediate-acting NPH insulin component). A summary of different types of insulin preparations can be seen in Table 3.1.

Insulin degludec

Currently available insulin analogs fail to completely mimic the physiological effects of basal insulin, especially at higher doses. Furthermore, lower doses do not achieve 24-hour insulin coverage in all individuals

Types of insulins and their pharmacokinetics

Type	Component	Names	Onset	Peak	Duration
Rapid	Bolus	Lispro	5–15 min	1–2 h	4–5 h
		Aspart			
		Glulisine			
Short	Bolus	Humulin S	30–60 min	2–3 h	6–8 h
		Actrapid			
Intermediate/ NPH	Basal	Insulatard	2–4 h	4–10 h	12–18 h
		Humulin I			
Long	Basal	Glargine	2–4 h	Flat	20–24 h
		Detemir	2 h	Broad	12–22 h
Premix	Basal	R + NPH 30/70	Onset, peak, and duration of action vary by component		
		Humulin M3, H			
		Mixtard 30 (withdrawn)			
		R + NPH 25/75			
		Insuman Combi 25			
		R + NPH 50/50			
		Insuman Combi 50			
Biphasic insulin analogs	Basal + bolus	Humalog Mix 25	Onset, peak, and duration of action vary by component		
		Humalog Mix 50			
		NovoMix 30			

Table 3.1 Types of insulins and their pharmacokinetics. NPH, neutral protamine hagedorn.

and there remains some within-subject variability with regards to the metabolic effect of insulin analogs, impeding optimal insulin titration.

Insulin degludec is a novel basal insulin analog that forms soluble multi-hexamers upon subcutaneous injection, resulting in an ultra-long action profile [3]. Insulin degludec has lower within-subject variability that insulin glargine [4]. Insulin degludec in patients with type 1 or type 2 diabetes improves long-term glycemic control with a lower rate of nocturnal hypoglycemia than insulin glargine, according to the results of recent Phase II trials (summarized in Table 3.2) [5–7].

In a Phase III study by Garber et al [8] involving 992 patients with type 2 diabetes comparing the efficacy and safety of degludec versus glargine over 1 year, insulin degludec use resulted in significantly lower rates of nocturnal hypoglycemia than insulin glargine (1.4 versus 1.8

Phase II trials of insulin degludec

Trial	Demographics	Duration	Treatment	Baseline HbA1c
Heise (2011)	178 insulin-naïve type 2 diabetes patients on 2 oral antidiabetic medications	16 weeks	IDegAsp (n=59)	8.3
			AF (n=59)	8.6
			IGlar (n=60)	8.4
Birkeland (2011)	178 patients with type 1 diabetes	16 weeks	IDeg(A) (n=59)	8.4
			IDeg(A) (n=60)	8.5
			IGlar (n=59)	8.3
Zinman (2011)	245 patients with type 2 diabetes on metformin	16 weeks	IDeg 3 times/wk (n=62)	8.8
			IDeg (group A) (n=60)	8.6
			IDeg (group B) (n=61)	8.8
			IGlar (n=62)	8.7

Table 3.2 Phase II trials of insulin degludec. AF, alternative formulation; HbA1c, glycated hemoglobin; IDeg, insulin degludec; IGlar, insulin glargine. Data adapted from [5–7].

episodes/patient-year; P=0.0399), with a non-significant difference in HbA1c at the end of 1 year. A similar study by Heller et al [9] compared insulin degludec with insulin glargine (once-daily) as a basal bolus treatment with insulin aspart over 1 year in 629 patients with type 1 diabetes, HbA1c was reduced by 0.4% in both groups, with a shorter time to titration target in the insulin degludec group (median 5 weeks versus 10 weeks; P=0.002). Rates of confirmed nocturnal hypoglycemia were also lower with insulin degludec than with insulin glargine (4.4 versus 5.9 episodes/patient-year; P=0.021).

Furthermore, Meneghini et al found that insulin degludec can be flexibly administered within 8 to 40 hours of the previous dose without compromising glycemic control [10]. The authors of this study claim this is particularly important for patients who need flexibility for personal (eg, sleeping in, going out late at night) or professional reasons (eg, shift

Treatment end point: HbA1c reduction	Treatment end point: hypoglycemia rate (events/patient year)	Treatment end point: nocturnal hypoglycemic events
↓1.3	1.2	1
↓1.5	2.4	27
↓1.3	0.7	3
↓0.57	47.9	5.1
↓0.54	59.5	8.8
↓0.62	66.2	12.3
↓1.5	2.3	4
↓1.3	0.6	2
↓1.3	0.9	1
↓1.5	1.1	0

work, night workers). The authors of this study are optimistic that the dosing flexibility could drive improved patient adherence, and potentially also improve long-term glucose control.

Pharmacokinetics of insulin

Insulin administered via subcutaneous injection is absorbed directly into the bloodstream. There is variability in insulin absorption at the various injection sites (eg, abdomen, deltoid, gluteus, thigh) due to differences in blood flow. Table 3.3 gives details of the factors affecting insulin absorption. Circulating insulin is distributed in equilibrium between free insulin and insulin bound to immuoglobulin G (IgG) antibodies. The kidneys and liver account for the majority of insulin degredation. Normally, the liver degrades approximately 60% of insulin released by the pancreas (via portal vein blood flow), while the kidneys degrade the

Factors affecting insulin absorption

Factor	Comment
Exercising injected area	Strenuous exercise of a limb within 1 hour of injection increases absorption. Clinically significant for regular human insulin
Local massage	Rubbing or massaging the injection site increases absorption
Temperature	Heat can increase absorption rate. Sauna, shower, or a hot bath should be avoided soon after injection. Cold temperatures have the opposite effect
Site of injection	Insulin is absorbed faster from the abdomen. (Clinically less relevant with analog insulins)
Lipohypertrophy	Injection into areas of lipohypertrophy delays insulin absorption
Jet injectors	Injectors increase absorption rate
Insulin mixtures	Absorption rates are unpredictable when suspension insulins are not adequately mixed (ie, they need to be resuspended)
Insulin dose	Larger doses have a delay in action and increased duration
Physical status (soluble versus suspension)	Suspension insulins must be sufficiently resuspended prior to injection to reduce variability

Table 3.3 Factors affecting insulin absorption.

remaining 35–45% [11]. However, when insulin is injected exogenously, the degradation profile is altered because insulin is no longer delivered via the portal vein. In this situation, the kidney has a greater role and degrades approximately 60% of insulin, with the liver degrading 30–40%.

Types of insulin regimens

There are a variety of insulin regimens, each of which should be tailored to meet the needs of the individual patient. The treatment option chosen should reflect the type of diabetes, the person's lifestyle, their age, their ability to self monitor glucose, the presence of obesity, and the individual's choice of pen device. The goal of therapy is an insulin profile that is as similar to the normal physiological state as possible.

Once-daily intermediate-acting or basal insulin, in combination with oral therapies, is the simplest sufficient regime for many elderly patients with type 2 diabetes. Given at breakfast or bedtime, this regimen could be used as an introduction to insulin after the failure of maximal oral therapy (with or without glucagon-like peptide-1 [GLP-1] analogs).

Twice-daily intermediate-acting or basal insulin is a simple regimen that can be used as an introduction to insulin therapy in type 2 diabetes, with the aim of moderate control of glycemia.

The aforementioned two regimens are not suitable for type 1 diabetes.

Twice-daily regimen with pre-mixed insulins or biphasic analogs is a very popular regimen and often used in the treatment of both type 1 and 2 diabetes. It can be very restrictive due to the fixed proportion of short and intermediate-acting insulin in the mixture but is often preferred by patients due to the convenience of requiring just two injections per day. This works well with patients that have regular meal habits and fixed carbohydrate content in their diet; however, if a patient's diet is variable and lifestyle is erratic, basal bolus is a better option. Advantages and disadvantages of the twice-daily premixed insulin regimen are summarized in Table 3.4.

Multiple daily insulin injections mimics endogenous insulin secretory profiles with a long-acting insulin that is administered once daily, along with rapid-acting insulin analogs (lispro, aspart, or glulisine) administered at each meal. Traditionally, basal bolus regimens were flawed because of the use of soluble insulin, which needed to be injected 30 minutes before a meal. However, with the advent of analogs, the bolus insulin can be taken just before the meal starts. In this regime, basal insulins can be either long-acting analogs (glargine, detemir) or isophane insulins (Insulatard, Humulin I). Advantages and disadvantages of basal bolus regimen are summarized in Table 3.5.

Advantages and disadvantages of premixed insulin	
Advantages	**Disadvantages**
Only two injections a day	Unexpected time-action profiles
	Unpredictable peaks
	Unpredictable glucose fluctuations
	Hypoglycemia is more common
	Difficult titrations
	Greater weight gain

Table 3.4 Advantages and disadvantages of premixed insulin.

Advantages and disadvantages of basal bolus regimen	
Advantages	**Disadvantages**
Higher flexibility, which is useful for: • erratic lifestyles • variable carbohydrate intake between meals • patients with suboptimal glycemic control with other regimens Dosing can be easily adjusted	Requires an average of four injections per day

Table 3.5 Advantages and disadvantages of basal bolus regimen.

Determining whether insulin is needed

Insulin is life-sustaining in patients with type 1 diabetes. Insulin replacement therapy is also essential for many individuals with genetic defects in insulin secretion, women with gestational diabetes when optimal glycemic control cannot be achieved with diet and exercise alone, and in a large percentage of individuals with type 2 diabetes when acceptable levels of glucose control cannot be achieved with oral agents or non-insulin secretagogues. There is now increasing evidence to support early use of insulin to achieve euglycemia, resulting in long-term sustained remission [12,13]. In addition, research showing an increased risk of complications with previous hyperglycemia [14] further underpins the importance of improving the 'metabolic memory.' Indications for insulin are listed in Table 3.6.

Insulin for type 1 diabetes

The Diabetes Control and Complication Trial (DCCT) showed that intensive insulin therapy (four injections or more per day or the use of an insulin

Indications for insulin
• Type 1 diabetes • Type 2 diabetes poorly controlled on maximal oral therapy ± GLP-1 analogs • Type 2 diabetes with contraindications to OHAs (eg, renal failure, poor tolerance) • Pregnancy • Post-acute myocardial infarction • Acute illness/infection • Perioperative period • Steroid-induced hyperglycemia • Total/partial pancreatectomy • Pancreatitis/pancreatic carcinoma

Table 3.6 Indications for insulin. GLP, glucagon-like peptide; OHA, oral hypoglycemic agent.

pump) significantly improves glycemic control over a sustained period compared with conventional insulin therapy (two injections per day) [15,16]. However, in this trial there was a comprehensive patient support element, which included diet, exercise plans and monthly visits with healthcare teams, making it difficult to separate the benefits of intensive insulin therapy from the benefits of having such intensive support. Therefore, intensive insulin therapy should be delivered as part of a comprehensive support package.

For adults with type 1 diabetes, an intensified treatment regimen should include either regular human insulin or rapid-acting analog insulin as the bolus insulin before meals, and NPH or basal analogs as the basal component of the regimen. Basal insulin analogs are recommended by the Scottish Intercollegiate Guideline Network in adults with type 1 diabetes who are experiencing severe or nocturnal hypoglycemia and are using an intensified insulin regimen [17].

Although the use of rapid acting analog insulin has a small but statistically significant effect in patients with type 1 diabetes (HbA1c reduction of 0.1%) when compared with regular human insulin, this is not clinically significant in the context of long-term complications. However, some studies have reported a reduction in hypoglycemia in association with analog insulin use [18,19]. Use of analog insulins is also associated with an improvement in treatment satisfaction scores [20].

Two meta-analyses have compared basal insulin analogs (glargine and detemir) and NPH insulin in adults with type 1 diabetes. The first meta-analysis, undertaken by the Canadian Agency for Drugs and Technologies in Health, concluded that the use of glargine was associated with a reduction in HbA1c of 0.11%, whereas use of detemir was associated with a 0.06% reduction in HbA1c [21]. In this analysis, there was no significant reduction in severe or nocturnal hypoglycemia with glargine use, whereas detemir use was associated with reductions in severe (response rate [RR] 0.74; 95% CI, 0.58–0.96) and nocturnal (RR 0.92; 95% CI, 0.85–0.98) hypoglycemia, though there was no reduction in overall hypoglycemia.

In a further meta-analysis comparing basal insulin analogs with NPH insulin, the mean reduction in HbA1c associated with the use of analogs was 0.07% [22]. From the evidence so far, detemir use was associated with significantly less weight gain when compared to NPH (0.26 kg/m^2; 95% CI, 0.06–0.47), although equivalent data were not available for glargine. One study included in the meta-analysis showed greater patient satisfaction, though no change in health-related quality of life was reported with the use of insulin glargine when compared with NPH. Therefore, while basal insulin analogs do not appear to offer clinically significant improvement in glycemic control, they may offer reductions in severe and nocturnal hypoglycemia. Insulin detemir may be associated with less weight gain than NPH insulin, but for optimal glycemic control, many individuals will require twice daily dosing.

Continuous subcutaneous insulin infusion (CSII) therapy is associated with modest improvements in glycemic control and should be considered for patients unable to achieve their glycemic targets [23]. CSII therapy should also be considered in patients who experience recurring episodes of severe hypoglycemia [23]. Using CSII therapy requires considerable input on the part of health care providers, especially from nurse specialists and dieticians, in addition to the purchase of a pump and consumables.

Although a number of meta-analyses have evaluated pump therapy, the randomized controlled trials (RCTs) in this area have been of poor quality despite being performed in specialized pump centers. Additionally, most of the RCTs were funded by pump companies and there is a lack of independently funded studies for comparison. Where patients have been selected for pump therapy on the basis of severe hypoglycemia, there is a three-fold lower rate of hypoglycemia associated with the institution of pump therapy (RR=2.89) [24]. In a 2008 meta-analysis [24], six RCTs were combined and there was an overall HbA1c reduction of 0.6% (6.6 mmol/mol) in patients treated with CSII therapy.

Insulin for type 2 diabetes

In type 2 diabetes, insulin is conventionally introduced when other therapies fail, although excellent glycemic control has been reported when insulin is initiated as first-line therapy when diet and lifestyle measures are ineffective [25]. However, the United Kingdom Prospective Diabetes Study (UKPDS) study did not show superior glycemic control or health related quality of life when insulin is used as an initial treatment [26]. Therefore, it is recommended to initiate therapy with oral agents and then proceed to insulin if the treatment goal is not achieved. The aim of insulin supplementation is glycemic control and a reduction in microvascular disease and, if possible, macrovascular disease, without inducing hypoglycemia or weight gain (Table 3.7).

However, insulin can be considered as an initial therapy for patients with type 2 diabetes, particularly in patients presenting with HbA1c >10% (86 mmol/mol), fasting plasma glucose >13.9 mmol/L (250 mg/dL), random glucose levels consistently >16.7 mmol/L (300 mg/dL) or ketonuria. Subsequent modifications can be made according to blood glucose and HbA1c values.

Insulin initiation: choosing a regimen

There have been two major studies looking at insulin initiation strategies for type 2 patients with diabetes on maximal oral therapy: A Trial comparing Lantus algorithms to Achieve Normal blood glucose Targets in subjects with Uncontrolled blood Sugar (AT.LANTUS) and Treating To Target in type 2 diabetes (4T) [27,28]. The AT.LANTUS study was a prospective, multicenter, 24-week randomized trial of 4961 suboptimally controlled type 2 subjects with diabetes (algorithm 1: $n=2493$; algorithm 2: $n=2468$). The algorithms used in the AT.LANTUS study are shown in Table 3.8. This study showed that glargine is safe and effective in improving glycemic control in a large, diverse population with long-standing type 2 diabetes [27]. A simple subject-administered titration algorithm conferred significantly improved glycemic control with a low incidence of severe hypoglycemia when compared with physician-managed titrations.

Evidence for insulin initiation

- effective in combination with oral agents;
- significantly lowers HbA1c;
- requires smaller dose of insulin;
- less weight gain (except in combination with thiazolidinediones);
- lower hypoglycemia with basal regimens.

Table 3.7 Evidence for insulin initiation. HbA1c, glycated hemoglobin.

Algorithms for insulin titration in the AT.LANTUS study

Mean FBG for the previous 3 consecutive days	Increase in daily basal insulin glargine dose (U)*	
	Algorithm 1[†]: titration at every visit; physician-driven	Algorithm 2[†]: titration every 3 days; subject-driven and reviewed by physicians at each visit
Starting dose	10 UI/day	Numerically equivalent to FBG in preceding 7 days (eg, FBG = 12 mmol/L, insulin dose = 12 UI/day)
≥100 and <120 mg/dL (≥5.6 and <6.7 mmol/L)	0–2 (at the discretion of the investigator)[‡]	0–2 (at the discretion of the investigator)[‡]
≥120 and <140 mg/dL (≥6.7 and <7.8 mmol/L)	2	2
≥140 and <180 mg/dL (≥7.8 and <10 mmol/L)	4	2
≥180 mg/dL (≥10 mmol/L)	6–8 (at the discretion of the investigator)[‡]	2

Table 3.8 Algorithms for insulin titration in the AT.LANTUS study. FBG, fasting blood glucose. *Target FBG ≤100 mg/dL (≤5.5 mmol/L). [†]Reviewed by physician at each visit, either in person or over the telephone; titration occured only in the absence of blood glucose levels <72 mg/dL) (<4.0 mmol/L). [‡]Magnitude of daily basal dose was at the discretion of the investigator.

In a post-hoc subanalysis [29] of an insulin-naive subpopulation of the AT.LANTUS study, in which glargine was initiated in suboptimally controlled type 2 diabetes patients on oral antidiabetic drugs (OAD), incidence of severe hypoglycemia was <1% and HbA1c decreased significantly between baseline and endpoint for patients receiving glargine plus 1 OAD (overall: –1.4%, P<0.001; algorithm 1: –1.3%; algorithm 2: –1.5%; P<0.03) and glargine plus >1 OAD (overall: –1.7%, P<0.001; algorithm 1: –1.5%; algorithm 2: –1.8%; P<0.001; [algorithm 1 versus algorithm 2]) (Table 3.9) [29]. This study demonstrated a greater reduction in HbA1c in patients randomized to the patient-driven algorithm (algorithm 2) treated with at least one OAD.

The 4T study [28] compared three different insulin strategies and provides an evidence base to guide the addition of insulin to OAD and glycemic control intensification in clinical practice [24]. In this multicenter study, 708 patients who had inadequate glycemic control while receiving metformin and sulfonylurea were randomly assigned to receive prandial insulin (once daily), detemir, or biphasic aspart 30 (twice daily) during the first year. Starting with the second year, sulfonylureas were replaced by an additional type of insulin if the patient's HbA1c level exceeded 6.5%.

Incidence of hypoglycemia in AT.LANTUS study					
	Insulin glargine + 1 OAD (n=316)			Insulin glargine + >1 OAD (n=499)		
	Algorithm 1 (n=170)	Algorithm 2 (n=146)	P	Algorithm 1 (n=256)	Algorithm 2 (n=243)	P
Severe hypoglycemia (% <2.8 mmol/L)	0	0	N/S	<1	<1	N/S
Symptomatic hypoglycemia (%)	13.5	15.1	N/S	18.8	16	N/S
Nocturnal hypoglycemia (%)	<1	2.1	N/S	2.7	4.5	N/S

Table 3.9 Incidence of hypoglycemia in AT.LANTUS study. OAD, oral antidiabetic agent; N/S, non-significant. Reprinted with permission from Davies et al [29].

Basal insulin was added to the prandial regimen, prandial insulin was added three-times daily to the basal regimen, and prandial insulin was added at midday to the biphasic regimen. Important aspects of this study are the three year duration and the aim of standardizing insulin regimens.

Median HbA1c levels at the end of three years were 7.1% in the biphasic group, 6.8% in the prandial group, and 6.9% in the basal group (P=0.28) [28]. A higher percentage of patients (44% in prandial group and 43% in basal group) had an HbA1c level of <6.5% when compared with the biphasic group (31.9%) [28]. Rates of hypoglycemia were lowest in the basal group (1.7%) and highest in the prandial group (5.7%) [28]. This trial shows that reasonable levels of glycemic control can be achieved with a low rate of major hypoglycemia, particularly when initiated with basal insulin [28]. Results of the 4T study are shown in Figure 3.3.

There is a striking difference in the results at the end of the first and third years of the 4T study. Although the basal regimen was the least successful in the first year, it was the most effective after three years, possibly because the insulin dose progressively increased. Similarly, the lower success rate of the biphasic regimen was probably due to the use of daily insulin doses below 1 unit/kg of body weight, which may be inadequate for improving insulin resistance. The ratios of prandial to basal insulin suggest that the use of increased doses of prandial insulin contributed to the efficacy of basal plus prandial regimens. Results also support the initial addition of basal insulin to oral therapy, with

Results of the 4T study

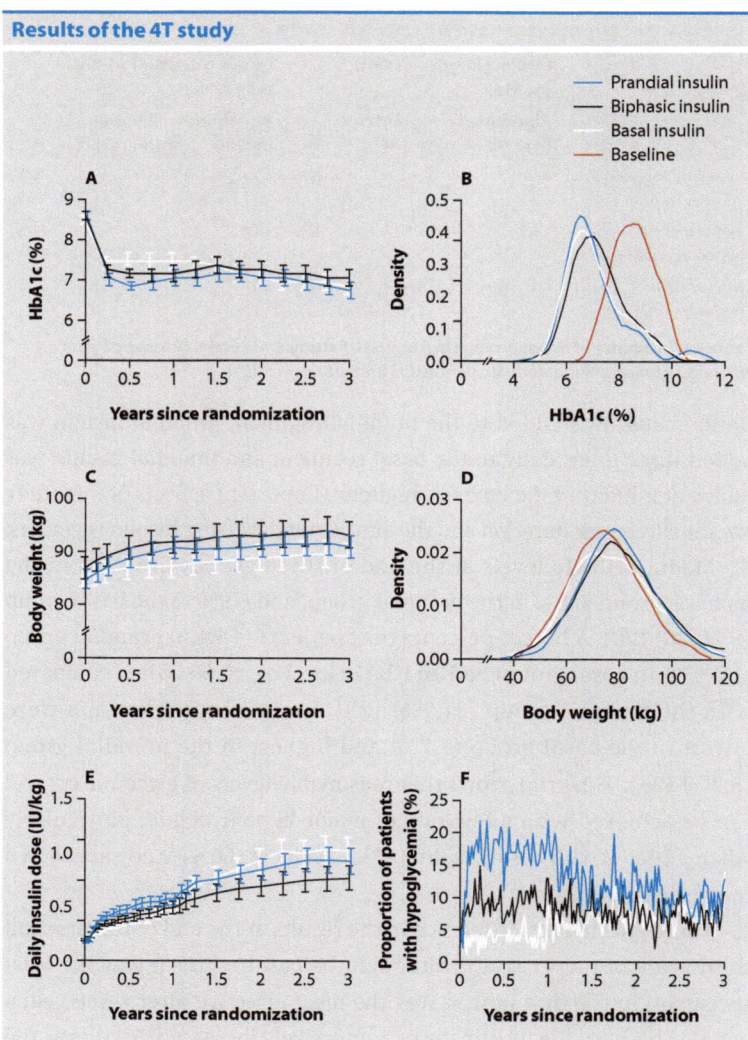

Figure 3.3 Results of the 4T study. Panel A shows median levels of glycated hemoglobin (HbA1c) in the three study groups, with a kernel-density plot of the distribution of values for patients in each group at 3 years, as compared with the distribution of values for all patients at baseline, shown in Panel B. Panel C shows mean body weight, with a kernel-density plot of the distribution of values for patients in each group at 3 years, as compared with the distribution of values for all patients at baseline, shown in Panel D. Panel E shows median insulin doses. Panel F shows the proportions of patients in the three study groups reporting grade 2 or grade 3 hypoglycemic events over time. The I bars indicate 95% confidence intervals. Reproduced with permission from Holman et al [28].

subsequent intensification to a basal-prandial regimen. Comparison of HbA1c, hypoglycemia, and body weight at the end of the first and third years in the 4T study is shown in Figure 3.4.

However, it should be noted that this study only used analog insulins. Regular human insulin is considered the first choice in consensus statements [30]. There is not sufficient evidence to determine the superiority of insulin analogs with respect to glucose control, endpoints, or costs.

Recommendations

Intensive insulin therapy, which utilizes basal insulin with multiple pre-meal injections of rapidly acting insulin, has become standard therapy in type 1 diabetes, although simpler regimens are often still used in type 2 diabetes. For example, twice-daily premixed insulin is not ideal

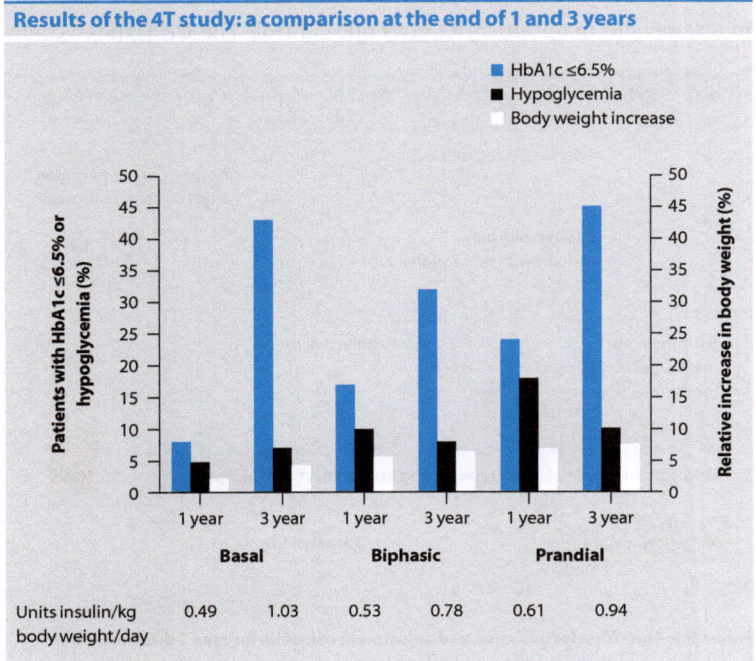

Figure 3.4 Results of the 4T study: A comparison at the end of 1 and 3 years. Shown are the proportions of patients who had a glycated hemoglobin (HbA1c) level of 6.5% or less or who had grade 2 or 3 hypoglycemia and the relative increase from baseline in body weight after the first year and the third year of the 4T study. Reproduced with permission from Holman et al [28].

for type 1 diabetes but it is a reasonable option for patients with type 2 diabetes who are doing well on a stable, fixed ratio.

If insulin is to be added to oral hypoglycemic therapy in patients with type 2 diabetes, basal insulin preparations should be included first. Sequential insulin strategies are found in Figure 3.5 [7].

Insulin can be considered initial therapy for all patients with type 2 diabetes, particularly patients presenting with HbA1c >10–12%, elevated plasma glucose >16.7–19.4 mmol/L (>300–350 mg/dL), or ketonuria. Subsequent modifications can be made according to blood glucose and HbA1c values [7].

Revisiting hypoglycemia

Hypoglycemia is a common, unpredictable, and potentially dangerous side effect of diabetes therapy. It remains the single greatest limitation in attempts to maintain strict glycemic control. The UK Hypoglycemia

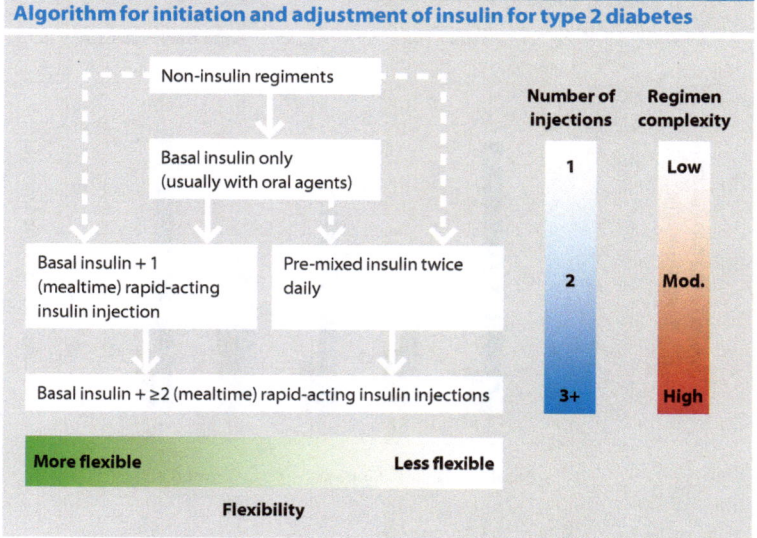

Figure 3.5 Algorithm for initiation and adjustment of insulin for type 2 diabetes. Basal insulin alone is generally the optimal initial regimen, and can be prescribed alongside non-insulin agent(s). If this does not adequately lower HbA1c, consider proceeding to basal plus mealtime insulin (1–3 injections). In patients with ≥9% HbA1c, twice-daily premixed insulin or an advanced basal plus mealtime insulin regimine can be considered (dashed line). Adapted with permission from Inzucchi et al [30].

Study Group has demonstrated that severe hypoglycemia is a common problem in insulin-treated type 2 diabetes and that the incidence increases with duration of insulin therapy [31] (Figure 3.6).

This study also demonstrated that the long disease duration group (>15 years) of type 1 diabetes patients experienced the highest frequency of severe hypoglycemic episodes (prevalence 46%, mean rate of 3.2 episodes per subject year). The mean rate in this study was substantially higher than that reported during the DCCT and is comparable with those observed in patients with hypoglycemia unawareness. This study also emphasizes that rates of hypoglycemia are often higher in unselected populations than in those in clinical trials and that even type 1 diabetes patients with a long duration who do not report unawareness remain vulnerable to severe episodes of hypoglycemia (due to failure of hypoglycemic counterregulation). The estimated percentage of severe hypoglycemic events in recent studies is shown in Figure 3.7 [32].

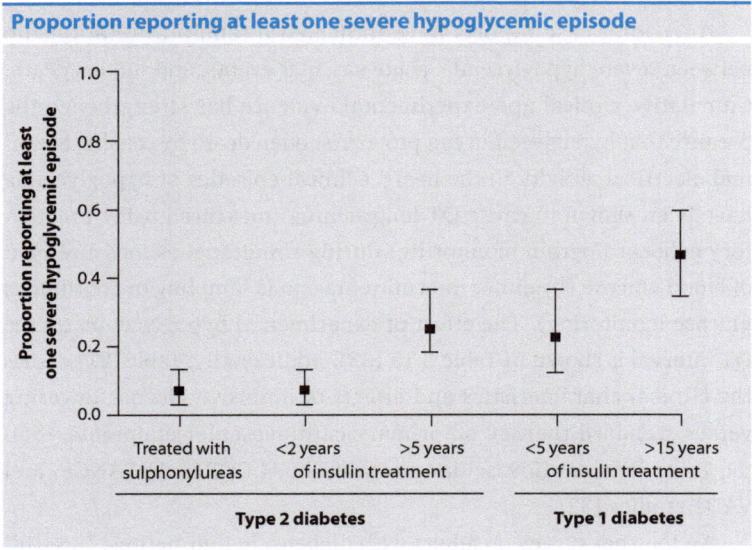

Figure 3.6 Proprotion reporting at least one severe hypoglycemic episode. For people with type 2 diabetes within the first 2 years of insulin therapy, rates of hypoglycemia were no higher than patients taking sulfonylureas and were much lower than in patients with type 1 diabetes. This effect seems to persist for at least a year. However, for type 2 patients on insulin for more than 5 years, the prevalence of mild and severe hypoglycemia was similar to that of type 1 diabetic patients with short duration. Reproduced with permission from the UK Hypoglycaemia Study Group [31].

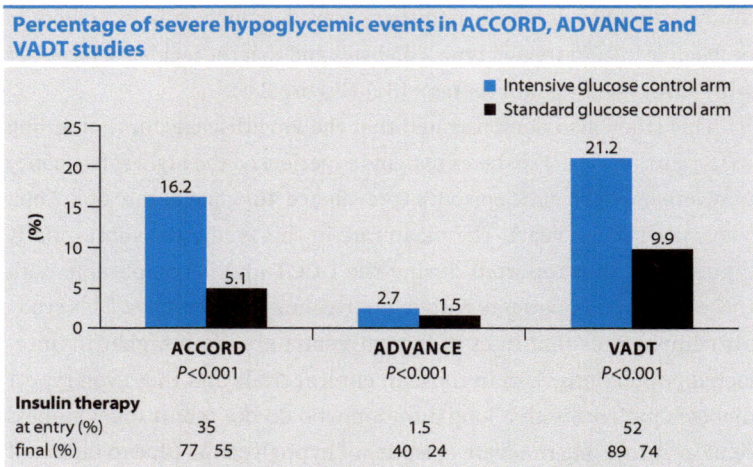

Percentage of severe hypoglycemic events in ACCORD, ADVANCE and VADT studies

Figure 3.7 **Percentage of severe hypoglycemic events in ACCORD, ADVANCE and VADT studies.** In all these trials, severe hypoglycemia was significantly higher in the intensive glucose-lowering arms compared with the standard arms. Reproduced with permission from Frier et al [32].

Anecdotal case reports have indicated a temporal relationship between severe hypoglycemia, acute vascular events, and sudden death. Cumulative clinical and experimental evidence has strengthened the premise that hypoglycemia can provoke sudden death by causing abnormal electrical activity in the heart. Clinical episodes of hypoglycemia have been shown to cause QT lengthening (measured using ambulatory echocardiogram monitoring) during simultaneous measurement of blood glucose (by either intermittent venous sampling or continuous glucose monitoring). The effect of experimental hypoglycemia on the QT interval is shown in Table 3.10 [33]. Additionally, Table 3.11 shows the clinical characteristics and effects of intensive glucose lowering versus standard therapy on primary cardiovascular endpoints, total mortality, and cardiovascular mortality in ACCORD, ADVANCE, and VADT studies [32].

An internet survey on adults with diabetes in four nations (US, UK, Germany, and France) that investigated the effect of non-severe nocturnal hypoglycemic events on diabetes management, sleep quality, and next-day function, found that following a nocturnal hypoglycemic event, 22.7% of subjects arrived late or missed work, 31.8% missed a meeting

The effect of experimental hypoglycemia on QT interval

Variable	Experiment	Baseline (Time 0)	End of clamp (Time 150 min)	Baseline versus end P
Mean QT interval	–GLIB	392 [24]	438 [41]	0.0003
	+GLIB	395 [32]	451 [33]	<0.0001
	Euglyc	392 [28]	393 [24]	NS
Mean QTc interval	–GLIB	430 [14]	491 [47]	0.0002
	+GLIB	443 [26]	506 [50]	0.0010
	Euglyc	427 [22]	438 [19]	NS
QT dispersion	–GLIB	34 [11]	104 [46	<0.0001
	+ GLIB*	44 [24]	116 [53]	0.0002
	Euglyc	30 [11]	30 [12]	NS
QTc dispersion	–GLIB	37 [12]	118 [53]	0.0001
	+GLIB*		49 [26]	131 [61]
	Euglyc	33 [13]	34 [14]	NS

*QT and QTc dispersion at baseline +GLIB are skewed, as one patient had a prolonged QT dispersion already at baseline

Median and range for these parameters are therefore also presented here:
QT dispersion, +GLIB baseline, median: 33, range: 22–105
QTc dispersion, +GLIB baseline, median: 35, range: 26–121

Table 3.10 The effect of experimental hypoglycemia on QT interval. Altered ventricular repolarisation during hypoglycemia in patients with type 2 diabetes mellitus. Euglyc, euglycemia; GLIB, glibenclamide. Reproduced with permission from Landstedt-Hallin et al [33].

Clinical characteristics and effects of intensive glucose lowering on cardiovascular outcomes in ACCORD, ADVANCE, and VADT studies

	ACCORD	ADVANCE	VADT
n	10,251	11,140	1,791
Age (years)	62	66	60
Men/women (%)	61/39	58/42	97/3
Duration of study (years)	3.5	5.0	5.6
BMI (kg/m^2)	32.2 ± 5.5	28.0 ± 5.0	31.3 ± 3.5
Duration of diabetes (years)	10	8	11.5
CVD	35%	32%	40%
Primary CVD end point	↓10% (P = 0.16)	↓6% (P = 0.37)	↓13% (P = 0.12)
Mortality (overall)	↑22% (P = 0.04)	↓7% (P = NS)	↑6.5% (P = NS)
CV mortality	↑35% (P = 0.02)	↓12% (P = NS)	↑25% (P = NS)

Table 3.11 Clinical characteristics and effects of intensive glucose lowering on cardiovascular outcomes in ACCORD, ADVANCE, and VADT studies. Primary cardiovascular endpoints, total mortality, and CV mortality in ACCORD, ADVANCE and VADT studies. The ACCORD study was prematurely interrupted due to an excessive rate of death in the intensive therapy group. BMI, body mass index; CV, cardiovascular; CVD, cardiovascular disease; NS, not significant. Reproduced with permission from Frier et al [32].

or deadline, and an average of 14.7 hours of work were lost [34]. In fact, it is estimated that the annual cost of hospitalization and ambulances for severe hypoglycemia in the UK is approximately £15 million [35].

Revisiting continuous glucose monitoring

Until recently, the evidence that continuous glucose monitoring (CGM) protects against hypoglycemic episodes was lacking. A recent study by Batellino et al [36] provided support for a reduced frequency of hypoglycemia with CGM. In this randomized, controlled multicenter study of 120 patients with type 1 diabetes, participants on intensive therapy were randomly assigned to receive real-time CMG or home monitoring with a blood glucose meter and wear a continuous glucose monitor every second week for five days. The primary outcome was time spent experiencing hypoglycemia and was significantly shorter in the CGM group when compared with the control group (mean time of 0.48 versus 0.97 hours/day, respectively) with a ratio of means of 0.49 (95% CI, 0.26–0.76; P=0.03). There was also significant reduction in the HbA1c in the CGM group [36].

In Vigersky et al, a RCT of 100 adults with type 2 diabetes who were not on prandial insulin compared the effects of 12 weeks of intermittent real time CGM (RT-CGM) with self-monitoring of blood glucose (SMBG) on glycemic control over a 40-week follow-up period [37]. The results showed a significant difference in HbA1c in the RT-CMG group at the end of 3 months active intervention (P=0.04), which was sustained during the follow-up period (Figure 3.8). The authors concluded that these 52-week data suggests a lasting effect on HbA1c from a short-term (ie, 12 weeks) exposure to RT-CGM and that it did so without any greater intensification of pharmacotherapy. Taking these trend data as a whole (continuous improvement until 24 weeks, with attenuation of the effect of RT-CGM thereafter although HbA1c does not return to baseline by 52 weeks), the authors concluded that periodic use of CGM technology might be beneficial [37]. Thus, CGM does have a role in improving glycemic control in select patient groups with diabetes but additional studies are will be needed to confirm cost-effectiveness.

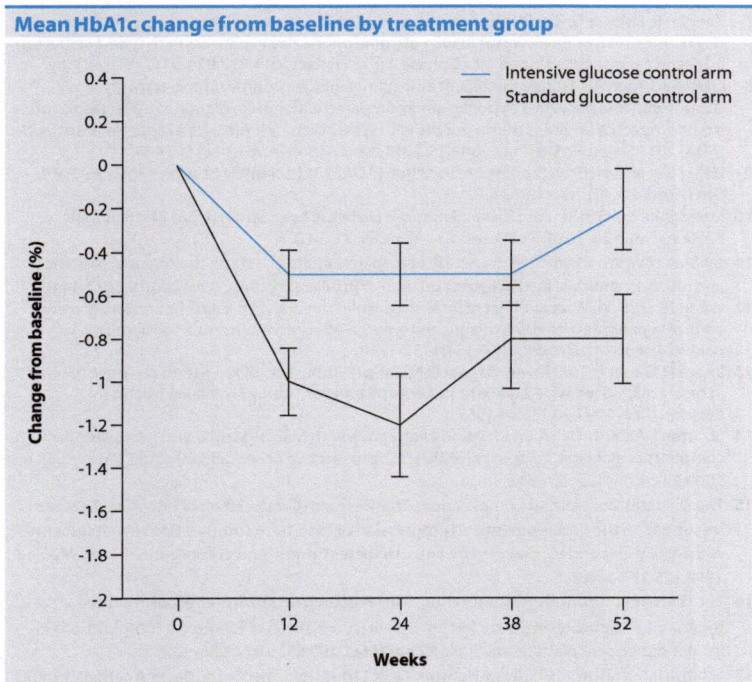

Mean HbA1c change from baseline by treatment group

Figure 3.8 Mean HbA1c change from baseline by treatment group. A decline in HbA1c over the course of the study differed between the groups net of other factors known to cause HbA1c change: age, sex, diabetes therapy, and initiation of insulin during the study. Specifically, the results of a multilevel model found that the decline for the SMBG group was 0.51% (*P*=0.002) and the decline for the RT-CGM group was 1.16% (*P*<0.0001). HbA1c, glycated hemoglobin. Reproduced with permission from Vigersky et al [37].

References

1   Andreas B. *Encyclopedia of Molecular Pharmacology*. Berlin: Springer; 2008.
2   Owens DR. New horizons - alternative routes for insulin therapy. *Nat Rev Drug Discov*. 2002;1:529-540.
3   Zinman B. Insulin degludec, a new generation ultra long-acting nsulin, used once daily or 3-times weekly in people with type 2 diabetes: comparison to insulin glargine (abstract). *Diabetes*. 2010;59 (suppl 1):A11.
4   Heise T. Insulin degludec: less pharmacodynamic variability than insulin glargine under steady state conditions (Abstract). *Diabetologia*. 2010;53(suppl.1):S387.
5   Heise T, Tack CJ, Cuddihy R, et al. A new-generation ultra-long-acting basal insulin with a bolus boost compared with insulin glargine in insulin-naïve people with type 2 diabetes: a randomized, controlled trial. *Diabetes Care*. 2011;34:669-674.
6   Birkeland KI, Home PD, Wendisch U, et al. Insulin degludec in type 1 diabetes: randomized controlled trial of a new-generation ultra-long-acting insulin compared with insulin glargine. *Diabetes Care*. 2011;34:661-665.

7   Zinman B, Fulcher G, Rao PV, et al. Insulin degludec, an ultra-long-acting basal insulin, once a day or three times a week versus insulin glargine once a day in patients with type 2 diabetes: a 16-week, randomised, open-label, phase 2 trial. *Lancet.* 2011;377:924-931.
8   Garber AJ, King AB, Francisco AMO, et al. Insulin degludec improves long-term glycemic control with less nocturnal hypoglycemia compared with insulin glargine: 1-year results from a randomized basal-bolus trial in people with type 2 diabetes; American Diabetes Association (ADA) 2011 Scientific Sessions; June 25, 2011; San Diego, CA. Abstract 0074-O.
9   Heller S et al. American Diabetes Association (ADA) 2011 Scientific Sessions; June 25, 2011; San Diego, CA. Abstract 0070-OR.
10 Meneghini L, Atkin SL, Bain S, et al. American Diabetes Association (ADA) 71st Scientific Sessions; June 25, 2011; San Diego, CA. Abstract 0035-LB.
11 ter Braak EW, Woodworth JR, Bianchi R, et al. Injection site effects on the pharmacokinetics and glucodynamics of insulin lispro and regular insulin. *Diabetes Care.* 1996;19:1437-1440.
12 Weng JP, Li YB, Xu W, et al. Effect of intensive insulin therapy on β-cell function and glycemic control in patients with newly diagnosed type 2 diabetes: a multicentre randomised parallel-group trial. *Lancet.* 2008;371:1753-1760.
13 Ilkova H, Glaser B, Tunckale A, Bagriacik N, Cerasi E. Induction of long-term glycemic control in newly diagnosed type 2 diabetic patients by transient intensive insulin treatment. *Diabetes Care.* 1997;20:1353-1356.
14 Stratton I, Adler A, Neil A. Association of glycemia with macrovascular and microvascular complications of type 2 diabetes (UKPDS 35): prospective observational study. *BMJ.* 2000;321:405-412.
15 The Diabetes Control and Complications Trial Research Group. Effect of intensive diabetes treatment on the development and progression of long-term complications in adolescents with insulin-dependent diabetes mellitus: Diabetes Control and Complications Trial. *J Pediatr.* 1994;125:177-188.
16 The Diabetes Control and Complications Trial Research Group. The effect of intensive treatment of diabetes on the development and progression of long-term complications in insulin-dependent diabetes mellitus. *N Engl J Med.* 1993;329:977-986.
17 Scottish Intercollegiate Guideline Network. SIGN 116: Management of diabetes: A national clinical guideline. SIGN website; 2010. www.sign.ac.uk/pdf/sign116.pdf. Accessed September 5, 2011.
18 Rosenstock J, Dailey G, Massi-Benedetti M, Fritsche A, Liz A, Saltman A. Reduced hypoglycemia risk with insulin glargine: a meta-analysis comparing insulin glargine with human NPH insulin in type 2 diabetes. *Diabetes Care.* 2005;28:950-955.
19 Heller SR, Amiel SA, Mansell P. Effect of the fast-action insulin analog lispro on the risk of nocturnal hypoglycemia during intensified insulin therapy. UK Lispro Study Group. *Diabetes Care.* 1999;22:1607-1611.
20 Bott U, Ebrahim S, Hirschberger S, Skovlund SE. Effect of the rapid-acting insulin analogue insulin aspart on quality of life and treatment satisfaction in patients with Type 1 Diabetes. *Diabet Med.* 2003;20:626-634.
21 Canadian Agency for Drugs and Technologies in Health (CADTH). Long-acting insulin analogs for the treatment of diabetes mellitus: meta-analyses of clinical outcomes. CADTH website. www.cadth.ca/en/products/health-technology-assessment/publication/757. Accessed September 5, 2011.
22 Monami M, Marchionni N, Mannucci E. Long-acting insulin analogs vs. NPH human insulin in type 1 diabetes. A meta-analysis. *Diabetes Obes Metab.* 2009;11:372-378.
23 Pickup JC. Management of diabetes mellitus: is the pump mightier than the pen? *Nat Rev Endocrinol.* 2012. [Epub ahead of print].
24 Pickup JC, Sutton AJ. Severe hypoglycemia and glycemic control in type 1 diabetes: meta-analysis of multiple daily insulin injections compared with continuous subcutaneous insulin infusion. *Diabet Med.* 2008;25:765-774.
25 Li YB, Xu W, Liao ZH, et al. Induction of long-term glycemic control in newly diagnosed type 2 diabetic patients is associated with improvement of β-cell function. *Diabetes Care.* 2004;27:2597-2602.

26 UK Prospective Diabetes Study (UKPDS) Group. Intensive blood glucose control with sulphonylureas or insulin compared with conventional treatment and risk of complication in patients with type 2 diabetes (UKPDS). *Lancet*. 1998;352:837-853.

27 Davies M, Storms F, Shutler S, Gomis R; for the AT.LANTUS Study Group. Improvement of glycemic control in subjects with poorly controlled type 2 diabetes - comparison of two treatment algorithms using insulin glargine. *Diabetes Care*. 2005;28:1282-1288.

28 Holman RR, Farmer AJ, Davies MJ, et al. Three-year efficacy of complex insulin regimens in type 2 diabetes. *N Engl J Med*. 2009;361:1736-1747.

29 Davies M, Lavelle-Gonzalez F, Storms F, Gomis R; for the AT.LANTUS Study Group. Initiation of insulin glargine therapy in type 2 diabetes subjects suboptimally controlled on oral antidiabetic agents: results from the AT.LANTUS trial. *Diabetes Obes Metab*. 2008;10:387-399.

30 Inzucchi SE, Bergenstal RM, Buse JB, et al. Management of hyperglycaemia in type 2 diabetes: a patient-centered approach. Position statement of the American Diabetes Association (ADA) and the European Association for the Study of Diabetes (EASD). *Diabetologia*. 2012;55:1577-1596.

31 UK Hypoglycaemia Study Group. Risk of hypoglycemia in types 1 and 2 diabetes: effects of treatment modalities and their duration. *Diabetologia*. 2007;50:1140-1147.

32 Frier B, Schernthaner G, Heller S. Hypoglycemia and cardiovascular risks. *Diabetes Care*. 2011;34(suppl 2):S132-S137.

33 Landstedt-Hallin L, Englund A, Adamson U, Lins PE. Increased QT dispersion during hypoglycemia in patients with type 2 diabetes mellitus. *J Intern Med*. 1999;246:299-307.

34 Brod M, Christensen T, Thomsen T, Bushnell DM. The impact of non-severe hyproglycemia events on work productivity and diabetes management. *Value Health*. 2011;14:665-671.

35 Battelino T, Phillip M, Bratina N, Nimri R, Oskarsson P, Bolinder J. Effect of continuous glucose monitoring on hypoglycemia in type 1 diabetes. *Diabetes Care*. 2011;34:705-800.

36 Hammer M, Lammert M, Mejias SM, Kern W. Costs of managing severe hypoglycemia in three countries. *J Med Econ*. 2009;281:290.

37 Vigersky RA, Fonda SJ, Chellappa M, Walker MS, Ehrhardt NM. Short- and long-term effects of real-time continuous glucose monitoring in patients with type 2 diabetes. *Diabetes Care*. 2012.

Chapter 4

Non-insulin agents for diabetes

Gayatri Sreemantula and Santosh Shankarnarayan

A variety of oral medications are available to treat type 2 diabetes and play an important role in maximizing blood glucose control and minimizing morbidity and mortality. These agents are summarized in Figure 4.1 and discussed individually in this chapter.

Metformin

Metformin is the only biguanide available in most parts of the world. Its major antihyperglycemic effect is reducing hepatic gluconeogenesis and increasing muscle glucose uptake by improving insulin sensitivity.

Metformin is the first-line therapy in treating overweight type 2 diabetes patients. It is also used in some insulin-treated overweight patients in order to reduce insulin requirements. As a monotherapy, metformin generally reduces glycated hemoglobin (HbA1c) by 1.5% [2,3]. In contrast with most antidiabetic drugs, metformin often leads to modest weight reduction or weight stabilization (although a 1 to 2 kg weight reduction is seen initially, the UK Prospective Diabetes Study [UKPDS] data suggests it does not significantly alter weight over a 10-year period [4]). During the post-interventional observation period of the UKPDS, reductions in the risk of macrovascular complications were maintained in the metformin group. A further advantage of metformin is the very low incidence of hypoglycemia.

J. Vora and M. Evans (eds.), *Managing Diabetes*,
DOI: 10.1007/978-1-908517-81-4_4, © Springer Healthcare 2012

Available oral antidiabetics

Drug class	Mechanism of action	Side effects
Metformin	Suppress hepatic glucose production (major)	GI side effects
	Improve insulin sensitivity in target tissues (minor)	Lactic acidosis (rare)
Sulfonylureas	Stimulate insulin secretion	Weight gain
		Hypoglycemia
Thiazolidinediones	Improve insulin sensitivity in target tissues	Weight gain
	Suppress hepatic glucose production (minor)	Edema
		Congestive heart failure
		Hepatoxicity
Alpha-glucosidase inhibitors	Delay carbohydrate absorption from the intestine	GI side effects
Meglitinides	Increase insulin secretion	Weight gain
		Hypoglycemia
Glucogon-like peptide-1 analogs	Augment insulin secretion	Nausea
	Supress glucagon	GI side effects
Dipeptidyl peptidase-4 inhibitors (gliptins)	Inhibit enzymatic degradation of endogenous incretin hormones	Nasopharyngitis
		Nausea

Figure 4.1 Available oral antidiabetics. GI, gastrointestinal. Adapted from Florez et al [1].

Characteristics of metformin:

- first-line therapy for overweight type 2 diabetes patients;
- reduces HbA1c by 1% to 2%;
- has a beneficial effect in overweight patients with regards to cardiovascular outcomes;
- slow titration minimizes gastrointestinal side effects;
- safe unless estimated glomerular filtration rate (eGFR)<30.

Glycemic control with metformin

In a Cochrane systematic review [5] that included 29 trials and compared metformin monotherapy with placebo, diet, or other oral agents, metformin showed a greater benefit with respect to stabilizing HbA1c and fasting blood glucose (FBG) when compared with placebo, with no significant change in body mass index, weight, lipid profile, or blood pressure (when compared with diet, metformin showed more benefit for HbA1c alone).

Additionally, participants using metformin showed marginally greater reductions in HbA1c compared with those using sulfonylureas. There was no significant difference in HbA1c between those using metformin and those using insulin, meglitinides, or alpha-glucosidase inhibitors.

In another systematic review [6] comparing the effectiveness and safety of oral medications for treating type 2 diabetes, second-generation sulfonylureas were associated with a trend towards greater HbA1c reduction compared with metformin, although this was not statistically significant.

In one observational study [7], metformin treatment failure occurred more rapidly in clinical practice than in clinical trials (42.0% vs 35.5%; mean failure rate of 17.0% per year). However, patients who initiated metformin within 3 months of diabetes diagnosis and patients who initiated metformin while the HbA1c was <7% failed at a much lower rate of 12.2% and 12.3% per year, respectively. This treatment failure after monotherapy with metformin requires the addition of other agents as combination therapy to optimize glycemic control.

Effect on cardiovascular morbidity

Among overweight patients (54% of whom were obese) in the UKPDS study [4], participants allocated to intensive glycemic control strategy with metformin (n=342) had a significant 32% relative risk reduction for any diabetes-related outcomes, 42% risk reduction for diabetes-related death, and 36% risk reduction for all-cause mortality compared with patients who received conventional care (primarily with diet alone; Figure 4.2A–D). The metformin group also had a 39% lower risk ($P=0.01$) of myocardial infarction than the conventional treatment group.

Side effects

Gastrointestinal side effects are common with metformin and therefore dose up-titration by 500 mg every week to the maximal tolerated dose is advised. Slow-release metformin is an option if gastrointestinal side effects cannot be tolerated (recommended dosage is up-titration of 500 mg every 2 weeks to a maximum of 2 g daily).

Renal dysfunction is the most common contraindication to the use of metformin. This is primarily due to the risk of lactic acidosis, a rare but

Results of the United Kingdom Prospective Diabetes Study 34

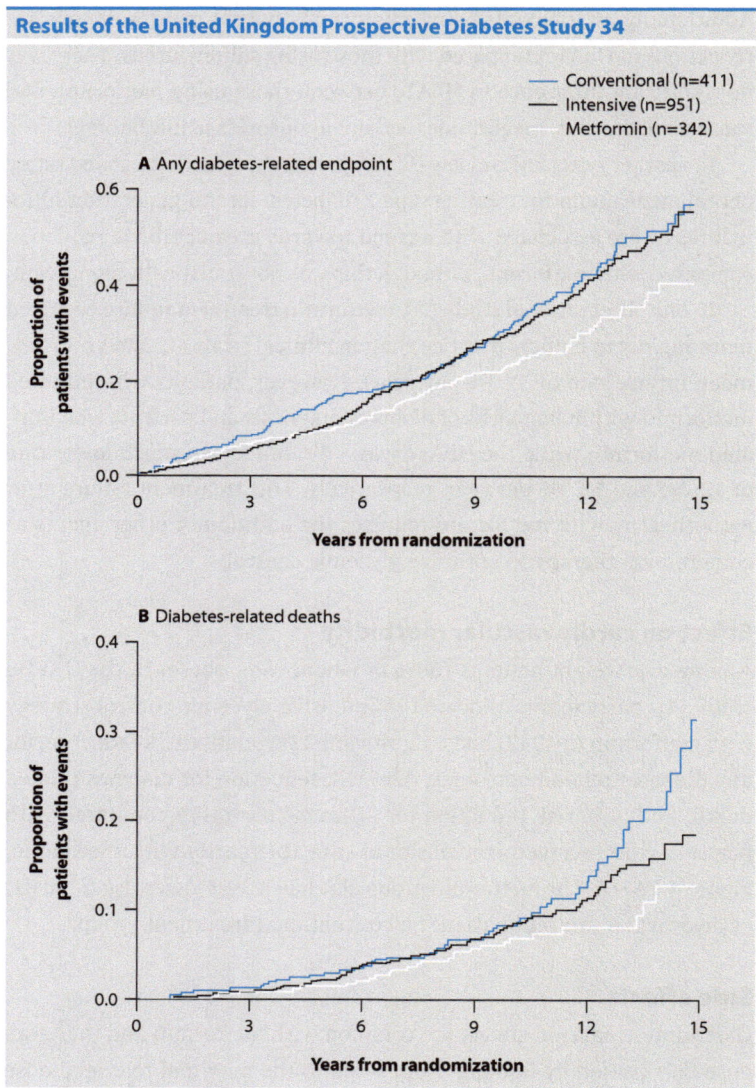

Figure 4.2 A–D Results of the United Kingdom Prospective Diabetes Study 34 (continues opposite).

Results of the United Kingdom Prospective Diabetes Study 34 (continued)

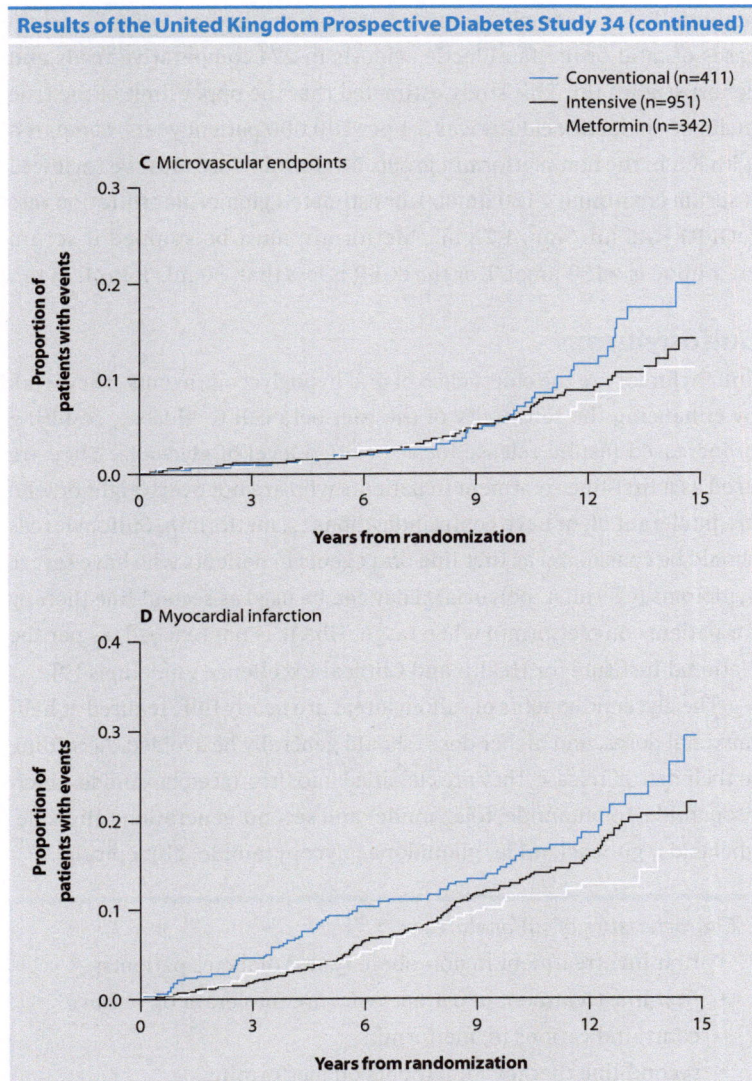

Figure 4.2 A–D Results of the United Kingdom Prospective Diabetes Study 34 (continued).
Kaplan-Meier plots in diet/metformin study for: A, any diabetes-related clinical endpoints;
B, diabetes-related deaths; C, microvascular endpoints; D, myocardial infarction. Intensive in this
figure indicates chloropropamide, glibenclamide, or insulin groups. Reproduced with permission
from Turner [4].

potentially fatal complication. A systematic review in 2006 found no cases of fatal or nonfatal lactic acidosis in 274 comparative trials and cohort studies [8]. This study estimated that the upper limit of the true incidence of lactic acidosis was 5.1 per 100,000 patient years, compared with 5.8 in the non-metformin group. Metformin dose must be reviewed if serum creatinine >130 μmol/L or estimated glomerular filtration rate (eGFR) <45 mL/min/1.73 m². Metformin must be stopped if serum creatinine is >150 μmol/L or the eGFR is less than 30 mL/min/1.73 m².

Sulfonylureas

Sulfonylureas are the oldest class of oral hypoglycemic agents. They work by enhancing the sensitivity of the islet beta cell to glucose, resulting in increased insulin release for a specified level of glycemia. They are used as a first-line treatment in patients who are not overweight or who are intolerant of, or have contraindications to, metformin. Sulfonylureas should be considered as first-line oral agents in patients who have severe symptoms (eg, thirst, polyuria). They can be used as second-line therapy for patients on metformin when target HbA1c is not reached, as per the National Institute for Health and Clinical Excellence guidelines [9].

The glycemic benefits of sulfonylureas are nearly fully realised at half-maximal doses, and higher doses should generally be avoided. According to their date of release, they are classified into first- (acetohexamide, chlor-propamide, tolbutamide, tolazamide) and second-generation (glipizide, gliclazide, glibenclamide, gliquidone, glycopyramide, glimepiride).

Characteristics of sulfonylureas:
- first-line treatment in non-obese type 2 diabetes patients;
- first-line treatment in patients who are intolerant of, or have contraindications to, metformin;
- second-line therapy for patients on metformin;
- improves HbA1c by 1.5% points;
- treats symptomatic hyperglycemia;
- increased risk of hypoglycemia;
- associated with weight gain.

Glycemic control with sulfonylureas

Sulfonylureas are moderately effective and can lower blood glucose concentrations by 1.5 to 3 mmol/L and HbA1c by 1.5% [10]. The glucose lowering potency of sulfonylureas is directly related to the initial glucose concentration at the outset of treatment, and is greater the higher the initial glucose concentration. In the UKPDS 33 study, the starting HbA1c concentration was around 9% and was lowered to about 7% by diet during the run-in period [10]. Adding sulfonlyureas further reduced HbA1c by 0.9%, compared with the diet-only group. The results of two systematic reviews investigating the effectiveness of oral diabetes therapies [5,6], when taken together, suggest that metformin and sulfonylureas have similar effects on HbA1c.

Modified-release glicalzide and glimepiride were shown to be equally effective at reducing HbA1c at 27 weeks, although there was no increased benefit of glimepiride versus the longer established glibenclamide at reducing HbA1c over 12–15 months [11].

Treatment with sulfonylureas results in the eventual loss of therapeutic effectiveness (secondary failure) in the range of 20–40%. In the UKPDS 33, 53% of newly diagnosed patients with diabetes treated with a sulfonylurea required the addition of insulin to maintain adequate glycemic control after 6 years [12].

Side effects

Concerns raised by the University Group Diabetes Program study in the 1970s that sulfonylureas as a drug class may increase cardiovascular risk in type 2 diabetes have not been substantiated by the UKPDS or the ADVANCE studies [10,12,13].

The major adverse effect of sulfonylureas is hypoglycemia (rate of 12.1% per annum with chlorpropamide in the UKPDS study). A Scottish population-based study [14] showed that 1 in every 100 patients with type 2 diabetes treated with a sulfonylurea experienced an episode of major hypoglycemia, compared with 1 in every 2000 treated with metformin and 1 in every 10 treated with insulin. Therefore, before beginning treatment with a sulphonylurea, the patient should be informed about the symptoms associated with and treatment of hypoglycemia. Long-acting sulfonylureas are more likely to cause hypoglycemia and therefore should be avoided, especially in older patients [15]. However, newer sulfonylureas have been found to cause less hypoglycemia [16].

Risk factors for hypoglycemia include increasing age, alcohol abuse, poor nutrition, and renal insufficiency. All sulfonylureas are associated with weight gain. The UKPDS 33 showed an average weight gain of 2.3 kg with the longer acting sulfonylureas [10]. They should be avoided in patients with porphyria.

Thiazolidinediones

Thiazolidinediones (TZDs) increase whole-body insulin sensitivity by activating nuclear receptors (peroxisome proliferator-activated recpetors; PPARs) and promoting esterification and storage of circulating free fatty acids in subcutaneous adipose tissue. Only pioglitazone is currently available in the UK following the suspension of rosiglitazone and its combinations in the EU. Rosiglitazone is a pure PPAR-gamma agonist, while pioglitazone also exerts some PPAR-alpha effects, which may account for the different effects they have on lipids.

Characteristics of thiazolidinediones:
- increased relative risk of myocardial infarction with rosiglitazone;
- rosiglitazone and its combinations are now suspended in the EU;
- increased risk of heart failure;
- associated with weight gain;
- increased risk of fractures.

Glycemic control with thiazolidinediones

The TZDs appear to have a more durable effect on glycemic control, particularly compared with sulfonylureas [16].

Side effects

In May 2007, safety concerns regarding TZDs attracted widespread attention with the publication of a meta-analysis by Nissen and Wolski suggesting that, compared with other treatments for diabetes, rosiglitazone was associated with a 43% higher risk of myocardial infarction ($P=0.03$)

and a 64% higher risk of cardiovascular death ($P=0.06$) [17]. Since then, subsequent reports have provided a relatively consistent message that rosiglitazone might indeed increase the risk of myocardial ischemic events (30–40% relative increase in risk), albeit with an inconsistent message regarding mortality [18,19].

However, the prospective pioglitazone clinical trial in macrovascular events (PROactive) study [20] demonstrated no significant effects of pioglitazone when compared with placebo on the primary cardiovascular disease (CVD) outcome after 3 years of follow-ups. Pioglitazone was associated with a 16% reduction in death, myocardial infarction, and stroke (a controversial secondary endpoint reported to have marginal statistical significance). In summary, meta-analyses have supported a possible beneficial effect of pioglitazone on CVD risk, although the data are less than conclusive for a CVD risk with rosiglitazone or a CVD benefit with pioglitazone [21].

Apart from these meta-analyses, several large-scale pharmacoepidemiologic investigations have used health care databases to provide 'real-world' data on the safety of TZDs. In studies in which TZDs drugs were compared, the results consistently showed that rosiglitazone was associated with greater risk of a CVD event than pioglitazone, or at best, the risks associated with these drugs were not statistically different [22] (Figure 4.3).

Amidst these controversies, the US Food and Drug Administration (FDA) and European Medicines Agency (EMA) have concluded that the benefits of TZDs outweigh the risks. The FDA has decided that rosiglitazone could remain available, but only under a very stringent restricted access program. However, in September 2010 the EMA recommended the suspension of marketing authorizations for all rosiglitazone-containing oral hypoglycemic medications licensed in the EU.

Other side effects associated with TZDs include the following:

- **Weight gain and fluid retention.** These are the most common adverse effects with TZDs, with weight gain varying from 1.5–5.3 kg [23]. The fluid retention may cause a two-fold increased risk of congestive heart failure when compared with a placebo [24]. There is an increase in adiposity (largely subcutaneous), with some reduction in visceral fat [25].

Incidence of time to event for acute myocardial infarction, stroke, heart failure, and all-cause mortality in elderly patients treated with rosiglitazone and pioglitazone

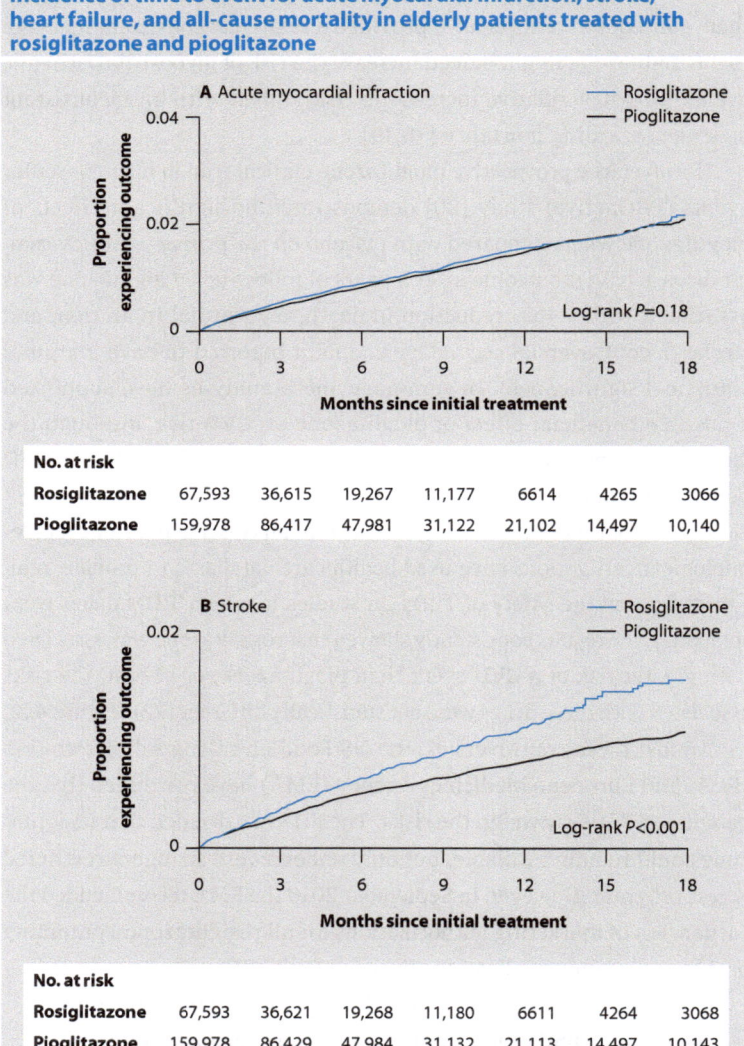

Figure 4.3 Incidence of time to event for acute myocardial infarction, stroke, heart failure, and all-cause mortality in elderly patients treated with rosiglitazone and pioglitazone (continues opposite).

Incidence of time to event for acute myocardial infarction, stroke, heart failure, and all-cause mortality in elderly patients treated with rosiglitazone and pioglitazone (continued)

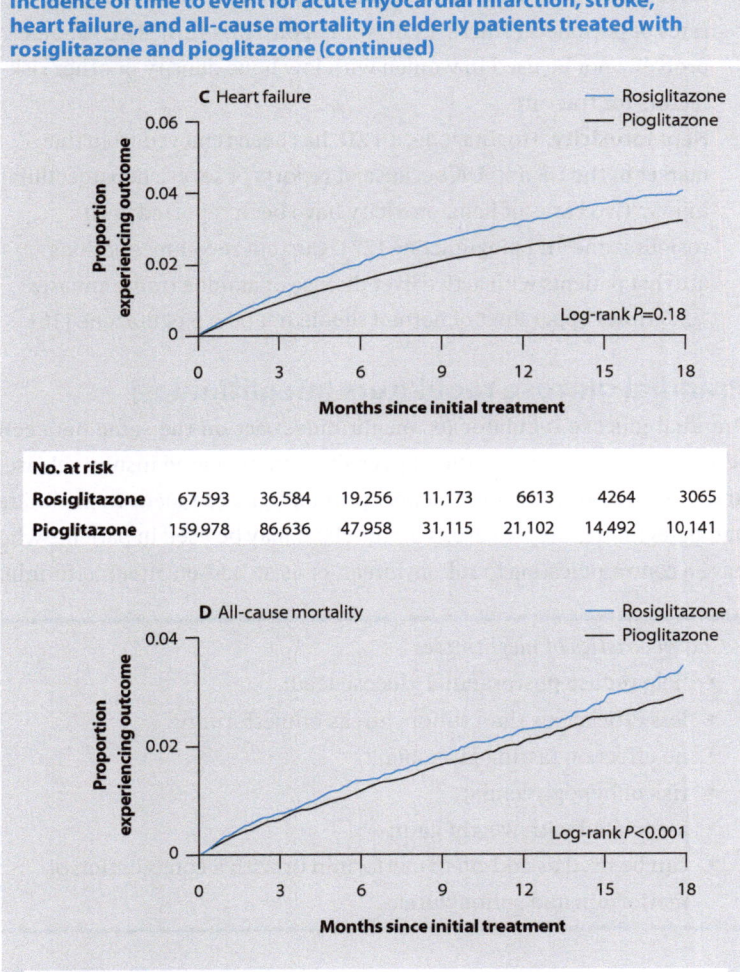

No. at risk

Rosiglitazone	67,593	36,584	19,256	11,173	6613	4264	3065
Pioglitazone	159,978	86,636	47,958	31,115	21,102	14,492	10,141

No. at risk

Rosiglitazone	67,593	36,638	19,277	11,183	6616	4266	3068
Pioglitazone	159,978	86,466	47,998	31,137	21,117	14,500	10,146

Figure 4.3 Incidence of time to event for acute myocardial infarction, stroke, heart failure, and all-cause mortality in elderly patients treated with rosiglitazone and pioglitazone (continued). These plots showed no difference in risk for acute myocardial infarction between rosigliatone and pioglitazone, but did show evidence of increased risk of stroke, heart failure, and death. Used with permission from Graham et al [22].

- **Increased fracture risk.** A meta-analysis in 2009 showed higher rates of peripheral fractures in women on TZDs [26]. TZDs should probably not be used in women with low bone density or other risk factors for fracture.
- **Hepatotoxicity.** Troglitazone, a TZD, has been removed from the market in the US and UK because of reports of severe hepatocellular injury. Two cases of hepatotoxicity have been reported with rosiglitazone and pioglitazone [27]. Current recommendations are that patients with active liver disease or alanine transaminases >2.5 times upper limit of normal should not take pioglitazone [16].

Prandial glucose regulators (meglitinides)

Prandial glucose regulator (or meglitinides) act on the same beta cell receptor as sulfonylureas, thereby resulting in increased insulin release, and are used for reducing the post-prandial glucose load. Repaglinide and nateglinide, the two drugs in this class, may be used in patients who have a contraindication to sulfonylureas, or as an add-on after metformin.

Characteristics of meglitinides
- help reduce postprandial glucose load;
- less efficacious than sulfonylureas or metformin;
- no effect on fasting glycemia;
- risk of hypoglycemia;
- associated with weight gain;
- can be used as add-on to metformin or with a combination of metformin and sulfonylureas.

Glycemic control with meglitinides

In a Cochrane review comparing meglitinides to placebo, both repaglinide and nateglinide resulted in improved glycemic control but produced a higher incidence of minor hypoglycemic events [28]. They generally provide better postprandial control. Repaglinide is more effective in lowering HbA1c than nateglinide and is principally metabolized by the liver. Therefore, it is safe to use in patients with renal impairment.

Side effects

Meglitinides cause less hypoglycemia than sulfonylureas, but the incidence of hypolglycemia is greater than that typically observed with metformin. However, the incidence of weight gain was greater (up to 3 kg in 3 months).

Alpha-glucosidase inhibitors

Alpha-glucosidase inhibitors (AGIs) are oral glucose-lowering agents that specifically inhibit alpha-glucosidases in the brush border of the small intestine [29]. These enzymes are essential for the release of glucose from more complex carbohydrates. The majority of the evidence base for AGIs (eg, acarbose) comes from their use as monotherapy in the management of patients with type 2 diabetes.

Characteristics of alpha-glucose inhibitors
- inhibits digestion of carbohydrates in the first half of the small intestine;
- can reduce HbA1c by 0.8%;
- can be used in combination with all oral hypoglycemics and insulin;
- use limited by gastrointestinal side effects;
- no risk of hypoglycemia;
- minimal effect on weight;
- may be useful in brittle diabetes.

Glycemic control with alpha-glucose inhibitors

One meta-analysis reported AGIs lowering HbA1c by 0.77% (8.7 mmol/mol; 95% CI, 0.9–0.6%) when compared with placebo [30]. AGIs inhibit postprandial glucose peaks, thereby leading to decreased post-load insulin levels, especially when compared with sulfonylureas. However, a small number of head-to-head trials and indirect data have shown that AGIs may be less efficacious in reducing HbA1c than other monotherapy regimens (AGI versus sulphonylurea: absolute reduction of 0.75% [8.20 mmol/mol]; 95% CI, 1.02–0.48) [31]. In another study, nocturnal hypoglycemia was shown to be prevented when an AGI was given before dinner [32]. Therefore, AGIs may be helpful in hard to control (or 'brittle') diabetes [33].

AGIs can be used in combination with nearly all established oral antidiabetics and insulin. In some cases of type 1 diabetes with a rapid postprandial glucose rise, and in cases of premeal hypoglycemia, AGIs can be introduced as an adjunct therapy.

Side effects
Side effects include abdominal pain, flatulence, and diarrhea. Side effects can be minimized by dose titration, starting with doses of 25 mg twice daily. The prevalence of gastrointestinal symptoms associated with AGIs (15–30%) is similar to that with metformin and higher than that with TZDs or sulfonylureas.

Contraindications
AGIs should not be given to patients with diverticulosis, large hernia, acute gastrointestinal disease, colitis, or inclusive and obstructive disease of the bowel due to their adverse effect on gas production. Other contraindications include pregnancy, lactation, and severe renal insufficiency.

Incretin-based therapies
The 'incretin effect', which was recognized as early as 1964, is demonstrated by the finding that an oral glucose load induces a greater insulin response compared with an intravenous infusion. The incretins are secreted by the enteroendocrine cells of the intestine in response to the ingestion of a meal. Apart from the enhanced insulin response, various other extra-pancreatic effects have been attributed to the incretins; they induce a delay in the gastric emptying, favor enhanced glycogen storage in the liver, and regulate satiety through their actions on the hypothalamic nuclei. These actions are helpful in regulating postprandial glucose and effectively mediate appetite reduction and weight loss. However, the rapid inactivation by the enzyme dipeptidyl peptidase-4 (DPP-4) within minutes of secretion restricts their biological activity. Two important incretin-based drug therapies have emerged to help overcome this hurdle: oral therapies that specifically inhibit the enzyme

DPP-4, and injectable preparations of DPP-4-resistant glucagon-like peptide-1 (GLP-1) analogs.

Glucagon-like peptide-1 analogs

The first GLP-1 analog introduced was exenatide; it was identified as a naturally occurring component of Gila monster saliva. Exenatide shares 53% structural homology to the human GLP-1 and is resistant to degradation by DPP-4. It augments insulin secretion from the pancreatic beta cells and suppresses glucagon secretion in a glucose-dependent manner. The insulin secretion subsides as the blood glucose approaches 4 mmol/L. Both the glucose-dependent insulinotropic and glucagonostatic effects help prevent the occurrence of hypoglycemia, unless exenatide is used in combination with other insulin secretogogues (especially sulfonylureas).

A meta-analysis [34] has reported an improvement in HbA1c of 1.01% (95% CI, -1.18 to -0.84) following 12 weeks of treatment with exenatide. As well as a sustained reduction in HbA1c, an average weight loss of 12 pounds was noticed over 2 years. In the absence of concomitant sulfonylurea therapy, there was no notable frequency of hypoglycemic events. Further trials have demonstrated similar reductions in HbA1c when exenatide was used in combination with other currently available antidiabetic agents such as metformin, sulfonylureas, TZDs, and insulin. A higher incidence of nausea, which is probably related to the delayed gastric emptying, has been the most common adverse event with exenatide. There have been reports of acute pancreatitis in 1 in 3000 exenatide users; although there is currently insufficient data to confirm a link, it is recommended that if a diagnosis of pancreatitis is confirmed exenatide use should be discontinued. Exenatide should not be used in patients with severe renal impairment (creatinine clearance <30 mL/minute) and in patients with moderate renal impairment (creatinine clearance 30 to 50 mL/minute). Monitoring of serum creatinine is warranted when exenatide is initiated and after dose titrations.

In the most recent update on the management of type 2 diabetes, NICE suggested that exenatide should be considered in patients who are very obese (body mass index ≥35) or in whom insulin is considered unacceptable because of occupational implications [9]. NICE also recommends that exenatide should only be continued if HbA1c is reduced by at least 1% and there is a weight loss of at least 3% of the initial body weight at 6 months [9]. Exenatide is usually started at 5 μg twice daily and titrated as required up to 10 μg twice daily after a month.

Following the approval of exenatide, newer molecules have been developed with improved pharmacokinetics. One example is liraglutide, a modified form of human GLP-1 with a palmitoyl fatty acid chain that prevents its degradation by DPP-4 and prolongs the half-life to 11–15 hours. It is injected once daily at a dose of 1.2 mg/day or 1.8 mg/day. Trials with liraglutide have demonstrated reductions of HbA1c of up to 1% (placebo subtracted) over 6 months when it is given as add-on therapy to metformin and/or sulfonylurea or a TZD [35]. Treatment with liraglutide was generally associated with weight reductions of approximately 2 or 3 kg. Liraglutide 1.8 mg/day has also been shown to significantly reduce HbA1c when compared to insulin glargine (1.33% versus 1.09%; 95% CI, 0.08–0.39; $P=0.0015$) [36]. Additionally, in a 26-week trial, significantly greater HbA1c reductions (0.33%) were seen with liraglutide when compared with twice-daily exenatide [36]. There were no occurrences of severe hypoglycemia with liraglutide treatment and nausea was generally transient.

Long-acting preparations of GLP-1 agonists such as exenatide long-acting release (LAR), which have a median half-life of 2 weeks, have been shown to have similar efficacy (eg, HbA1c reduction of 1.7%) and weight loss in patients treated with 2 mg doses [37]. Taspoglutide and albiglutide are examples of other GLP-1 agonists with weekly or less frequent dosing, and are now being evaluated in clinical trials. The clinical development of taspoglutide has been suspended pending clarification of immunogenicity issues. A nonpeptide GLP-1 receptor agonist is currently being developed that would offer an alternative with the convenience of oral administration.

Dipeptidyl peptidase-4 inhibitors (gliptins)

DPP-4 inhibitors (or gliptins) inhibit the enzymatic degradation of endogenous incretin hormones and restores them to physiological levels. They are conveniently administered as tablets and produce similar effects to GLP-1 analogs. Some of the gliptins now available in the UK include sitagliptin, vildagliptin, and saxagliptin.

Sitagliptin is taken once daily at a dose of 100 mg. In a 2006 clinical trial [38], sitagliptin reduced the mean HbA1c by about 0.7% and did not alter body weight or increase the incidence of hypoglycemia. Sitagliptin reduces 2-hour postprandial blood glucose by approximately 3 mmol/L.

Vildagliptin is a potent and selective dipeptidyl peptidase-4 inhibitor (DPP-4) that blocks dipeptidyl peptidase-4 inactivation of glucagon-like peptide-1 (GLP-1) and glucose dependent insulinotropic polypeptide (GIP) [39]. The drug has demonstrated efficacy when given as monotherapy or in combination with other antidiabetic drugs [40–42]. Vildagliptin is well tolerated and has a low risk of hypoglycemia and weight gain. Its efficacy when added to metformin [43] as well as its safety (overall [44], but also with respect to cardiovascular and cerebrovascular events [45] and adverse events of special interest [46]) has been thoroughly reviewed elsewhere, including in special populations such as the elderly [43–45].

In patients with moderate or severe renal impairment, vildagliptin (50 mg once daily) blocks DPP-4 activity over 24 hours (reflecting the increased exposure) and thus 50 mg once daily is the appropriate dose [44]. In these type of patients, vildagliptin added to ongoing antidiabetic therapy had a safety profile similar to placebo during 1-year observation. Furthermore, relative to placebo, a clinically significant decrease in HbA1c was maintained throughout 1-year treatment with vildagliptin [47]. Both sitagliptin and vildagliptin are metabolized mostly in the kidneys and hence if creatinine levels <50mL/min or in cases of advanced chronic kidney disease, dose reduction is necessary [7]. Nasopharyngitis, acute pancreatitis, and skin reactions are some of the other reported side effects with gliptins [48].

The ADA/EASD guidelines recommend that the gliptins can be added to metformin as second-line therapy [16]. They can also be used as third-line agents in combination with metformin plus sulfonylureas, TZDs, or insulin [16]. Recently, sitagliptin has been licensed for use with insulin and in patients with moderate or severe renal impairment with dose alterations.

Newer DPP-4 inhibitors include algogliptin and linagliptin. In the EU, linagliptin has been approved for use in combination with metformin and metformin plus sulphonylureas and is also approved as monotherapy in patients inadequately controlled by diet and exercise alone and for whom metformin is inappropriate or contraindicated. Linagliptin is predominately eliminated via nonrenal processes, making it suitable in patients with renal impairment. However, development of algoglipitin has been delayed, as the regulatory authorities felt exisiting clinical data did not meet cardiovascular safety requirements. However, the drug has now been resubmitted for consideration following a cardiovascular outcome study (EXAMINE), which sought to define the cardiovascular safety profile of algoglipitin in patients at high-risk for cardiovascular events [49].

Colesevelam

Colesevelam is a bile acid sequestrant (BAS) which has a well-defined role in lowering cholesterol. Reductions in both fasting and post-prandial glucose have been noted in studies with colesevelam [50]. Various mechanisms of action have been proposed but the most likely hypothesis is thought to be the deactivation of farsenoid X receptors by BAS, leading to an increase in liver X receptor (LXR) activity. The LXR is known to increase glucose uptake in muscle and adipose tissue and reduce hepatic gluconeogenesis. Also, colesevelam is thought to reduces both carbohydrate and fat absorption from the gut, resulting in weight loss and improvements in glycemic control. Reduction in the enterohepatic circulation of bile acids is thought to indirectly influence glucose metabolism.

Four prospective studies evaluating the effectiveness of colesevelam (used at a dose of 3.75 g/day) in patients with type 2 diabetes have shown a reduction in HbA1c by 0.50–0.54%, along with an average low density lipoprotein (LDL) cholesterol reduction of approximately 14.8% (Figure 4.4) (reviewed in [50]). Trials evaluating the benefit of colesevelam as an add-on to metformin or as an add-on to metformin plus other oral antidiabetic drug therapy demonstrated HbA1c reductions of 0.54% and 0.62% at the end of 26 weeks [51]. Similarly, another multi-center, randomized, placebo-controlled trial [52] evaluating the efficacy of adding colesevelam to baseline insulin monotherapy or insulin

Clinical trials of colesevelam treatment of diabetes mellitus

Trial	Demographics	Duration	Treatment	Baseline A1C	Treatment end point
Zieve (2007)	36 men; 29 women T2DM on metformin or sulfonylurea or both	12 weeks	Colesevelam HCL 3.75 g/day	7.9%	HbA1c: ↓ 0.50% FPG: ↓ 14.0 mg/dL* LDL-C: ↓ 11.7%
Bays (2008)	164 men; 152 women T2DM on metformin ± OAD	26 weeks	Colesevelam HCL 3.75 g/day	8.2%	HbA1c: ↓ 0.54% FPG: ↓ 13.9 mg/dL* LDL-C: ↓ 15.9%
Fonseca (2008)	250 men; 211 women T2DM on sulfonlyurea ± OAD	26 weeks	Colesevelam HCL 3.75 g/day	8.2%	HbA1c: ↓ 0.54% FPG: ↓ 13.5 mg/dL* LDL-C: ↓ 16.7%
Goldberg (2008)	148 men; 139 women T2DM on insulin ± OAD	16 weeks	Colesevelam HCL 3.75 g/day	8.3%	HbA1c: ↓ 0.50% FPG: ↓ 14.6 mg/dL* LDL-C: ↓ 12.8%

Figure 4.4 Clinical trials of colesevelam treatment of diabetes mellitus. *Not statistically significant. FPG, Fasting plasma glucose; HbA1c, Hemoglobin A1c; HCL, Hydrochloride; LDL-C, Low-density lipoprotein cholesterol; OAD, Oral antidiabetic agent; T2DM, type 2 diabetes mellitus; ↓, decrease.

plus other oral antidiabetic drugs demonstrated a HbA1c reduction of 0.59% ± 0.15 and 0.44 ± 0.12% at 16 weeks respectively ($P<0.001$).

Colesevelam has been specifically designed with a unique structure to improve tolerability and reduce potential drug interactions compared to older BAS compounds (eg, cholestyramine and colestipol). In human drug interaction studies [53] with colesevelam, no significant effect has been demonstrated on the bioavailability of many common drugs such as digoxin, fenofibrate, lovastatin, metoprolol, quinidine, valproic acid, warfarin, or statins. The most common adverse events reported with colesevelam include constipation, nasopharyngitis, dyspepsia, hypoglycemia, nausea, and hypertension.

In both Europe and the US, colesevelam is now indicated as adjuvant therapy to diet and exercise to reduce LDL cholesterol levels in patients inadequately controlled with statins. It has also been licensed for use in adults with type 2 diabetes to improve glycemic control. The established dual role of lowering both cholesterol and glucose makes colesevelam distinct from the other conventional oral antidiabetic drugs. Colesevelam will therefore offer another reasonable treatment choice for treating patients with type 2 diabetes.

Bromocriptine

Bromocriptine has been used in clinical practice for over 30 years as a treatment for hyperprolactinemia, galactorrhea, and parkinsonism. Based on its ability to modulate central glucose and energy metabolism pathways, a new indication for the use of bromocriptine in the treatment of diabetes was proposed [54].

In animal experiments with insulin-resistant models, attenuation of dopaminergic tone in the hypothalamus was associated with overstimulation of hepatic glucose production and adipose lipolysis, leading to increases in circulating glucose, free fatty acids, and triglycerides [55]. This is thought to contribute to peripheral insulin resistance and cause beta cell dysfunction via lipotoxicity and glucotoxicity. Timed-pulse administration of bromocriptine increases the dopaminergic tone and decreases the release of norepinephrine and serotonin [55], which are believed to reduce glucose intolerance and insulin resistance in peripheral tissues.

A new formulation of bromocriptine-quick release (QR) produces a short-duration pulse of bromocriptine within the circulation due to its rapid absorption when administered orally. In preclinical studies of patients with type 2 diabetes, the circadian resetting of the dopamine signal improved an array of metabolic derangements and restored the insulin sensitivity [55]. In Phase II and Phase III clinical trials, bromocriptine-QR was shown to reduce the HbA1c by 0.6%–1.2% (7–13 mmol/mol) both when used as a monotherapy and in combination with other antidiabetes medications (Figure 4.5) [54]. Modest reductions in blood pressure and triglyceride levels have been observed in these clinical trials with no increase in the risk for hypoglycemia or weight gain. In studies, bromocriptine-QR was administered at doses of 1.6–4.8 mg/day, and at these levels the drug has not been associated with retroperitoneal fibrosis or heart valve abnormalities.

The FDA has approved the use of bromocriptine in patients with type 2 diabetes as an adjunct to diet and exercise and as an add-on therapy to established oral agents or insulin. However, the FDA has stated that bromocriptine should not be used to treat type 1 diabetes or diabetic ketoacidosis, since there has been no demonstrable benefit for glycemic control in these patients.

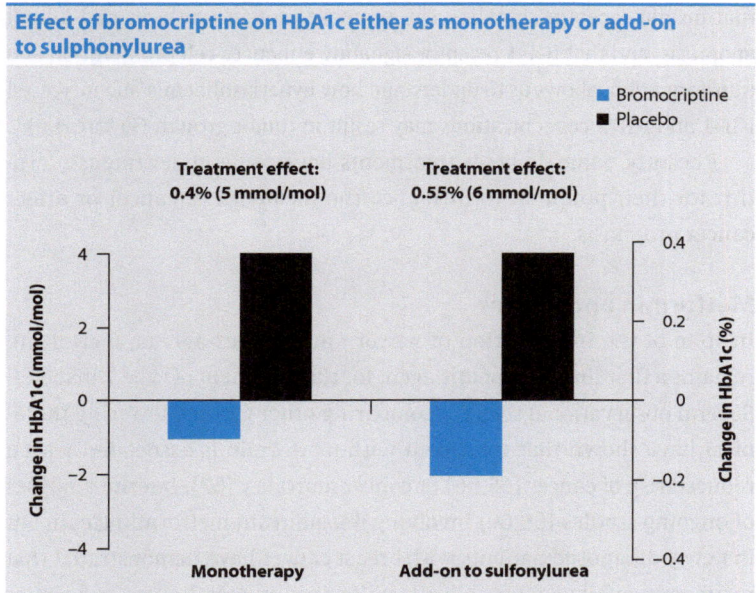

Figure 4.5 Effect of bromocriptine on HbA1c either as monotherapy or add-on to sulfonylurea. Reproduced with permission from Fonseca et al [52].

A noninsulin-dependent mechanism of action makes bromocriptine unique from the other agents that are currently in clinical use. Further studies are required to elucidate the exact mechanisms and biochemical effects of bromocriptine through which it may modulate central nervous system regulatory pathways of glucose and energy metabolism [55]. More information on the effects of adding bromocriptine to incretin-based therapies is also needed. Taken as a once daily preparation in the morning, bromocriptine will make a valuable treatment option both alone and as an add-on therapy to existing antidiabetic therapies that mainly target postprandial glucose levels.

Diabetes treatments: cancer risk and prognosis

Epidemiological studies [56–64] have reported that diabetes and obesity are linked to an increased risk of certain cancers (eg, hepatic, pancreatic, colon, endometrial, breast, bladder) in association with higher levels of insulin, C-peptide, and insulin-like growth factor 1 (IGF-1). Understanding that insulin receptor signaling can promote protein synthesis and inhibit apoptosis, and that IGF-1 receptor signaling enhances cell proliferation and transformation, allows us to understand how hyperinsulinemia and increased IGF-1 and IGF-2 concentrations may result in tumor growth (Figure 4.6).

Recently, some diabetes treatments have come under intense scrutiny for their potential to influence the incidence of cancer or affect cancer prognosis.

Metformin and cancer

In spite of the introduction of newer antidiabetes agents, metformin remains a first-line therapeutic agent for the treatment of type 2 diabetes. Several observational studies (comparing other glucose-lowering therapies) have shown that treatment with metformin is associated with a reduced risk of cancer [65,66] or cancer mortality [67]. Interim analyses of ongoing studies [68,69] involving neoadjuvant metformin treatment in newly diagnosed patients with breast cancer have demonstrated that metformin exhibits favorable effects on insulin metabolism and tumor cell proliferation and apoptosis (Figure 4.7).

Similar findings of higher cancer risk have been reported from observational studies among patients with type 2 diabetes treated with sulphonylureas [70]. However, due to the low incidence of cancer in these studies, further associations with specific cancer sites were not found and it was difficult to determine whether the findings reflected excess cancer among users of sulphonylureas. There have been no reports on the affect of meglitinides or incretin-based therapies on human cancer incidence.

Pioglitazone and bladder cancer risk

Although TZDs have recently been surrounded by controversy in regards to their potential impact on cardiovascular health, in vitro studies have shown that PPARγ agonists [71,72] appear to have several anticancer properties such as inhibition of cell growth, differentiation, and the ability to induce apoptosis. However, these findings are contradicted by increased tumorigenesis observed in rodent studies and the possibility of an increased risk of bladder cancer in human studies [73,74]. In April 2011, Piccini et al [75] concluded by using the Adverse Event

Signaling of insulin receptors and insulin-like growth factor 1

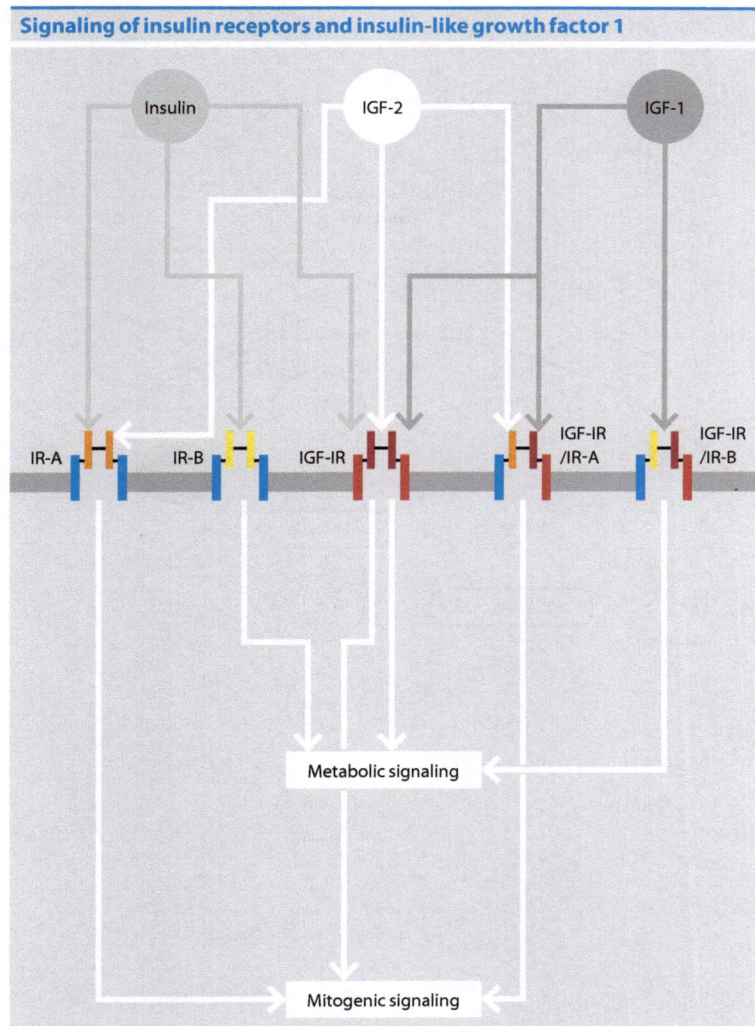

Figure 4.6 Signaling of insulin receptors and insulin-like growth factor 1. Figure depicts the insulin receptors (IR-A and IR-B), the insulin-like growth factor 1 receptor (IGF-1R), and the hybrid receptors (IGF-1R/IR-A and IGF-1R/IR-B). Insulin signals primarily through IR-A and IR-B with lower affinity for IGF-1R. IGF-1 binds to the IGF-1R and IGF-1R/IR-A and IGF-1R/IR-B hybrids. IGF-2 binds to the IR-A, IGF-1, and IGF-1R/IR-A hybrid receptor. Binding of insulin and IGF-2 to the IR-A results in mitogenic signaling. Activation of the IR-B receptor initiates metabolic signaling. IGF-1 and IGF-2 signaling through the IGF-1R mostly activates mitogenic signaling pathways, as does binding to the IGF-1R/IR-A hybrid. Activation of the IGF-1R/IR-B hybrid leads to predominantly metabolic effects. Reproduced with permission from Gallagher EJ et al [64].

Signaling of insulin receptors and insulin-like growth factor 1

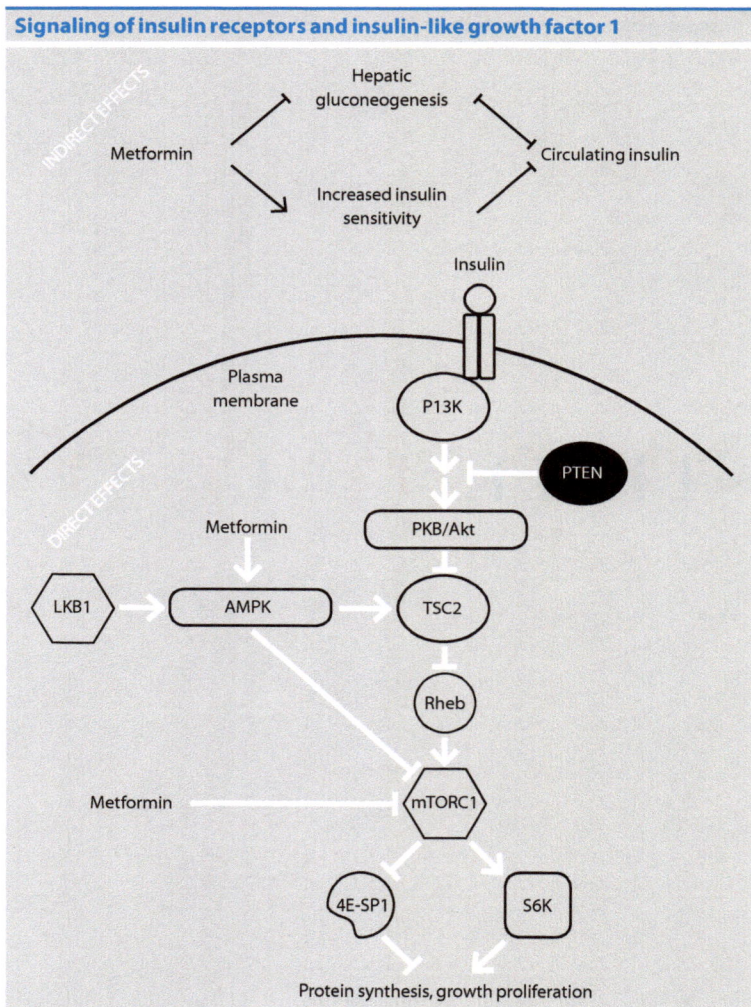

Figure 4.7 Direct and indirect effects of metformin on cancer. Metformin activates AMPK leading to stabilization of TSC2 and inhibition of mTORC1 signaling and protein synthesis. Metformin can also directly target mTORC1 independently of AMPK and TSC2. Systemically, metformin sensitizes tissues to insulin, reduces hepatic gluconeogenesis, and lowers circulating insulin levels, indirectly reducing receptor tyrosine kinase activation and PI3K signaling. AMPK, AMP-activated protein kinase; 4E-BP1, eukaryotic initiation factor 4E-binding protein-1; LKB1, liver kinase B1; mTORC1, mammalian target of rapamycin complex 1; PI3K, phosphatidylinositol-3-kinase; PKB/Akt, protein kinase B; PTEN, phosphatase and tensin homologue deleted on chromosome 10; Rheb, Ras homologue enriched in brain; S6K, ribosomal protein S6 kinase; TSC2, tuberous sclerosis complex 2. Reproduced with permission from Dowling et al [70].

Reporting System database that a significant risk of bladder cancer was associated with pioglitazone irrespective of treatment duration. In June 2011, the Food and Drug Administration (FDA) in the US warned that the use of pioglitazone for more than a year may be associated with an increased risk of bladder cancer [76]. The French and German regulatory bodies went on to suspend pioglitazone in the same month [77,78].

The FDA warning is based on a review of data from the first half of an ongoing 10-year epidemiological study [79]. This preliminary analysis showed that although pioglitazone was not associated with an overall increase in the risk of bladder cancer, there was a weak association with longer exposure and the highest cumulative dose of the drug [79]. The FDA's current advice is to avoid using pioglitazone in patients with active bladder cancer and to prescribe the drug with caution for patients with a prior history of bladder cancer, weighing the benefits of blood glucose control against the unknown risks for cancer recurrence.

After a recent thorough review [80] by the EMA Committee for Medicinal Products for Human Use (CHMP) of the benefits and risks of pioglitazone treatment, it is has been found that the benefits of the drug appear to outweigh the risks, with the CHMP stating that pioglitazone continues to be a valid option for treating certain patients with type 2 diabetes. It further clarified its position in a subsequent press release [81] by stating that pioglitazone is an option only when other treatments (eg, metformin) have not been deemed suitable or have failed to work adequately.

References

1   Florez H. Sanchez A, Marks J. Type 2 diabetes. In: *Diabetes in The Brain*. London: Springer; 2009.
2   Bailey CJ, Turner RC. Metformin. *N Engl J Med*. 1996;334:574-583.
3   DeFronzo R, Goodman A. Efficacy of metformin in patients with non-insulin-dependent diabetes mellitus. *N Engl J Med*. 1995;333:541-549.
4   Turner R. Effect of intensive blood-glucose control with metformin on complications in overweight patients with type 2 diabetes (UKPDS 34). *Lancet*. 1998;352:854-865.
5   Saenz A, Fernandez-Esteban I, Mataix A, Ausejo M, Roque M, Moher D. Metformin monotherapy for type 2 diabetes mellitus. *Cochrane Database Syst Rev*. 2005;(3):CD002966.
6   Bolen S, Wilson L, Vassy J, Feldman L, Yeh J, Marinopoulos S. Comparative effectiveness and safety of oral diabetes medications for adults with type 2 diabetes. Rockville, MD: Agency for Healthcare Research and Quality; 2007. www.effectivehealthcare.ahrq.gov/ehc/products/6/39/OralFullReport.pdf. Accessed September 5, 2012.
7   Brown JB, Connor C, Nichols GA. Secondary failure of metformin monotherapy in clinical practice. *Diabetes Care*. 2010;33:501-506.

8   Salpeter S, Greyber E, Pasternak G, Salpeter EE. Risk of fatal and nonfatal lactic acidosis with metformin use in type 2 diabetes mellitus. *Cochrane Database Syst Rev.* 2006;(1):CD002967

9   National Insititute for Health and Clinical Excellence. Type 2 diabetes NICE clinical guideline 87; 2009. www.nice.org.uk/CG87. Accessed September 5, 2012.

10 Turner R. Intensive blood-glucose control with sulfonylureas or insulin compared with conventional treatment and risk of complications in patients with type 2 diabetes (UKPDS 33). *Lancet.* 1998;352:837-853.

11 Schernthaner G, Grimaldi A, di Mario U, et al. GUIDE study: double-blind comparison of once-daily gliclazide MR and glimepiride in type 2 diabetic patients. *Eur J Clin Invest.* 2004;34:535-542.

12 Wright A, Burden AC, Paisey RB, et al; for the UK. Prospective Diabetes Study Group. Sulfonylurea inadequacy: efficacy of addition of insulin over 6 years in patients with type 2 diabetes in the UK Prospective Diabetes Study (UKPDS 57). *Diabetes Care.* 2002;25:330-336.

13 Patel A, MacMahon S, Chalmers J, et al; for the ADVANCE Collaborative Group. Intensive blood glucose control and vascular outcomes in patients with type 2 diabetes. *N Engl J Med.* 2008;358:2560-2572.

14 Leese GP, Wang J, Broomhall J, et al. Frequency of severe hypoglycemia requiring emergency treatment in type 1 and type 2 diabetes: a population-based study of health service resource use. *Diabetes Care.* 2003;26:1176-1180.

15 Shorr RI, Ray WA, Daugherty JR, Griffin MR. Individual sulfonylureas and serious hypoglycemia in older people. *J Am Geriatr Soc.* 1996;44:751-755.

16 Inzucchi SE, Bergenstal RM, Buse JB, et al. Management of hyperglycaemia in type 2 diabetes: a patient-centered approach. Position statement of the American Diabetes Association (ADA) and the European Association for the Study of Diabetes (EASD). *Diabetologia.* 2012;55:1577-1596.

17 Nissen SE, Wolski K. Effect of rosiglitazone on the risk of myocardial infarction and death from cardiovascular causes. *N Engl J Med.* 2010;304:411-418.

18 Singh S, Loke YK, Furberg CD. Long-term risk of cardiovascular events with rosiglitazone: a meta-analysis. *JAMA.* 2007;298:1189-1195.

19 Home PD, Pocock SJ, Beck-Nielsen H, et al. Rosiglitazone evaluated for cardiovascular outcomes in oral agent combination therapy for type 2 diabetes (RECORD): a multicentre, randomised, open-label trial. *Lancet.* 2009;373:2125-2135.

20 Dormandy JA, Charbonnel B, Eckland DJA, et al; for the PROactive investigators. Secondary prevention of macrovascular events in patients with type 2 diabetes in the PROactive Study (Prospective pioglitazone clinical trial in macrovascular events): a randomized controlled trial. *Lancet.* 2005;366:1279-1289.

21 Lincoff AM, Wolski K, Nicholls SJ, Nissen SE. Pioglitazone and risk of cardiovascular events in patients with type 2 diabetes mellitus: a meta-analysis of randomized trials. *JAMA.* 2007;298:1180-1188.

22 Graham DJ, Ouellet-Hellstrom R, Macurdy TE, et al. Risk of acute myocardial infarction, stroke, heart failure, and death in elderly medicare patients treated with rosiglitazone or pioglitazone. *JAMA.* 2010;304:411-418.

23 Yki-Jarvinen H. Thiazolidinediones. *N Eng J Med.* 2004;351:1106-1118.

24 Nissen SE, Nissen SE, Wolski K. Effect of rosglitazone on the risk of myocardial infarction and death from cardiovascular causes. *N Eng J Med. 2007*; 2457-2471.

25 Miyazaki Y, Mahankali A, Matsuda M, et al. Effect of pioglitazone on abdominal fat distribution and insulin sensitivity in type 2 diabetes patients. *J Clin Endocrinol Metab.* 2002;87:2784-2791.

26 Loke YK, Singh S, Furberg CD. Long-term use of thiazolidinediones and fractures in type 2 diabetes: a meta-analysis. *CMAJ.* 2009;180:32-39.

27 Scheen AT. Hepatotoxicity with thiazolidiones: is it a class effect? *Drug Saf.* 2001;12:873-888.

28 Black C, Donnelly P, McIntyre L, Royle PL, Shepherd JP, Thomas S. Meglitinide analogs for type 2 diabetes mellitus. Cochrane Database Syst Rev. 2007;(2):CD004654.

29 Bischoff H. Pharmacology of alpha-glucose inhibition. *Eur J Clin Invest.* 1994;24 (suppl 3):3-10.

30 van de Laar FA, Lucassen PL, Akkermans RP, van de Lisdonk EH, Rutten GE, van Weel C. Alpha-glucosidase inhibitors for patients with type 2 diabetes: results from a Cochrane systematic review and meta-analysis. *Diabetes Care.* 2005;28:154-163.

31 Bolen S, Wilson L, Vassy J, Marinopolous S. *Comparative effectiveness and safety of oral diabetes medications for adults with type 2 diabetes.* Rockville, MD: Agency for healthcare research and disability; 2007.

32 Taira M, Takasu N, Komiya I, Taira T, Tanaka H. Voglibose administration before the evening meal improves nocturnal hypoglycemia in insulin-dependent diabetic patients with intensive insulin therapy.*Metabolism.* 2000;4:440-443.

33 Hanefeld M. Alpha-glucose inhibitors. In: Goldstein BJ, Muller-Wieland D, eds. *Type 2 Diabetes: Principles and Practice.* Second edition. New York: Informa; 2008: 127.

34 Amori RE, Lau J, Pittas AG. Efficacy and safety of incretin therapy in type 2 diabetes: systematic review and meta-analysis. *JAMA.* 2007;298:194-206.

35 Lovshin, JA, Drucker, JD, et al. Incretin-based therapies for type 2 diabetes mellitus. *Nat. Rev. Endocrinol.* 2009;5:262-269.

36 Shyangdan DS, Royle P, Clar C, Sharma P, Waugh N, Snaith A. Glucagon-like peptide analogues for type 2 diabetes mellitus. *Cochrane Database Syst Rev.* 2011;(10):CD006423.

37 Kim D, MacConell L, Zhuang D, et al. Effects of once-weekly dosing of a long-acting release formation of exenatide on glucose control and body weight in subjects with type 2 diabetes. *Diabetes Care.* 2007;30:1487-1493.

38 Rosenstock J, Brazg R, Andryuk PJ, et al. Efficacy and safety of the dipeptidyl peptidase-4 inhibitor sitagliptin added to ongoing pioglitazone therapy in patients with type 2 diabetes: a 24-week, multicenter, randomized, double-blind, placebo-controlled, parallel-group study. *Clin Therapeutics.* 2006;28:1556-68.

39 Ahren B, Foley JE. The islet enhancer vildagliptin: mechanisms of improved glucose metabolism. *Int J Clin Pract Suppl.* 2008;159:8-14.

40 Keating GM. Vildagliptin: a review of its use in type 2 diabetes mellitus. *Drugs.* 2010;70:2089-2112.

41 Fonseca V, Baron M, Shao Q, Dejager S. Sustained efficacy and reduced hypoglycemia during one year of treatment with vildagliptin added to insulin in patients with type 2 diabetes mellitus. *Horm Metab Res.* 2008;40:427-430.

42 Matthews DR, Dejager S, Ahren B, et al. Vildagliptin add-on to metformin produces similar efficacy and reduced hypoglycaemic risk compared with glimepiride, with no weight gain: results from a 2-year study. *Diabetes Obes Metab.* 2010;12:780-789.

43 Halimi S, Raccah D, Schweizer A, Dejager S. Role of vildagliptin in managing type 2 diabetes mellitus in the elderly. *Curr Med Res Opin.* 2010;26:1647-1656.

44 Pratley RE, Rosenstock J, Pi-Sunyer FX, et al. Management of type 2 diabetes in treatment-naive elderly patients: benefits and risks of vildagliptin monotherapy. *Diabetes Care.* 2007;30:3017-3022.

45 Schweizer A, Dejager S, Foley JE, Shao Q, Kothny W. Clinical experience with vildagliptin in the management of type 2 diabetes in a patient population >75 years: a pooled analysis from a database of clinical trials. *Diabetes Obes Metab.* 2011;13:55-64.

46 Lukashevich V, Schweizer A, Shao Q, Groop PH, Kothny W. Safety and efficacy of vildagliptin versus placebo in patients with type 2 diabetes and moderate or severe renal impairment: A prospective 24-week randomized placebo-controlled trial. *Diabetes Obes Metab.* 2011;13:947-954.

47 Kothny W, Shao Q, Groop PH, Lukashevich V. One-year safety, tolerability and efficacy of vildagliptin in patients with type 2 diabetes and moderate or severe renal impairment. *Diabetes Obes Metab.* 2012; [Epub ahead of print].

48 Campbell RK, Cobble ME, Reid TS, Shomali ME. Safety tolerability and nonglycemia effects of incretin-based therapies. *J Fam Pract.* 2010;59(suppl 1): S20-S27.

49 White WB, Bakris GL, Bergenstal RM, et al. EXamination of cArdiovascular outcoMes with aloglIptIN versus standard of carE in patients with type 2 diabetes mellitus and acute coronary syndrome (EXAMINE): a cardiovascular safety study of the dipeptidyl peptidase 4 inhibitor alogliptin in patients with type 2 diabetes with acute coronary syndrome. *Am Heart J.* 2011;162:620-626.

50 Marrs JC. Colesevelam for the management of type 2 diabetes. *Expert Opin Drug Metab Toxicol.* 2009;5:187-194.

51 Fonseca VA, Rosenstock J, Wang AC, et al. Colesevelam HCl improves glycemic control and reduces LDL cholesterol in patients with inadequately controlled type 2 diabetes on sulfonylurea-based therapy. *Diabetes Care.* 2008;31:1479-1484.

52 Fonseca VA, Handelsman Y, Staels B. Colesevelam lowers glucose and lipid levels in type 2 diabetes: the clinical evidence. *Diabetes Obes Metab.* 2010;12:384-392.

53 Welchol product information – cholesevelam hydrochloride. 2007. www.welchol.com/pi/htm. Accessed May 22, 2012.

54 Holt RIG, Barnett AH, Bailey CJ, et al. Bromocriptine: old drug, new formulation and new indication. *Diabetes Obes Metab.* 2010;12:1048-1057.

55 Scranton R, Cincotta A. Bromocriptine – unique formulation of a dopamine agonist for the treatment of type 2 diabetes. *Expert Opin Pharmacother.* 2010;11:269-279.

56 Larsson SC, Orsini N, Brismar K, Wolk A. Diabetes mellitus and risk of bladder cancer: A meta-analysis. *Diabetologia.* 2006;49:2819-2823.

57 El-Serag HB, Hampel H, Javadi F. The association between diabetes and hepatocellular carcinoma: A systematic review of epidemiologic evidence. *Clin Gastroenterol Hepatol.* 2006;4:369-380.

58 Huxley R, Ansary-Moghaddam A, Berrington de González A, Barzi F, Woodward M. Type-II diabetes and pancreatic cancer: a meta-analysis of 36 studies. *Br J Cancer.* 2005;92:2076-2083.

59 Larsson SC, Orsini N, Wolk A. Diabetes mellitus and risk of colorectal cancer: A meta-analysis. *J Natl Cancer Inst.* 2005;97:1679-1687.

60 Mitri J, Castillo J, Pittas AG. Diabetes and risk of non-Hodgkin's lymphoma: A meta-analysis of observational studies. *Diabetes Care.* 2008;31:2391-2397.

61 Kasper JS, Giovannucci E. A meta-analysis of diabetes mellitus and the risk of prostate cancer. *Cancer Epidemiol Biomarkers Prev.* 2006;15:2056-2062.

62 Friberg E, Orsini N, Mantzoros CS, Wolk A. Diabetes mellitus and risk of endometrial cancer: A meta-analysis. *Diabetologia.* 2007;50:1365-1374.

63 Larsson SC, Mantzoros CS, Wolk A. Diabetes mellitus and risk of breast cancer: A meta-analysis. *Int J Cancer.* 2007;121:856-862.

64 Gallagher EJ, Fierz Y, Ferguson RD, LeRoith D. The pathway from diabetes and obesity to cancer: insulin and IGF-1 signalling. *Endocrine Practice.* 2010;16:864-873.

65 Monami M, Lamanna C, Balzi D, Marchionni N, Mannucci E: Sulphonylureas and cancer: a case-control study. *Acta Diabetol.* 2009;46:279-284.

66 Currie CJ, Poole CD, Gale EA. The influence of glucose-lowering therapies on cancer risk in type 2 diabetes. *Diabetologia.* 2009;52:1766-77.

67 Landman GW, Kleefstra N, van Hateren KJ, Groenier KH, Gans RO, Bilo HJ. Metformin associated with lower cancer mortality in type 2 diabetes: ZODIAC-16. *Diabetes Care.* 2010;33:322.

68 Niraula S, Stambolic V, Dowling RJO, et al. Clinical and biologic effects of metformin in early stage breast cancer. *Cancer Res.* 2010:70(Suppl 24):104S.

69 Hadad SM, Dewar JA, Elseedawy E et al. Gene Signature of metformin actions on primary breast cancer within a window of opportunity randomized clinical trial. *J Clin Oncol.* 2010;28(Suppl):560.

70 Dowling RJO, Goodwin PJ, Stambolic V. Understanding the benefit of metformin use in cancer treatment. *BMC Medicine.* 2011;9:33.

71 Elstner E, Muller C, Koshizuka K, et al. Ligands for peroxisome proliferator-activated receptor gamma and retinoic acid receptor inhibit growth and induce apoptosis of human breast cancer cells in vitro and in BNX mice. *Proc Natl Acad Sci. USA.* 1998;95:8806-8811.

72 Clay CE, Namen AM, Astumi G, et al. Magnitude of peroxisome proliferator-activated receptor-gamma activation is associated with important and seemingly opposite biological responses in breast cancer cells. *J. Investig. Med.* 2001;49:413-420.

73 Dormandy JA, Charbonnel B, Eckland DJ, et al; for the PROactive investigators. Secondary prevention of macrovascular events in patients with type 2 diabetes in the PROactive Study (PROspective pioglitAzone Clinical Trial In macroVascular Events): a randomised controlled trial. *Lancet.* 2005;366:1279-1289.

74 Dormandy J, Bhattacharya M, van Troostenburg de Bruyn AR. Safety and tolerability of pioglitazone in high-risk patients with type 2 diabetes: an overview of data from PROactive. *Drug Saf.* 2009;32:187-202.

75 Piccinni C, Motola D, Marchesini G, Poluzzi E. Assessing the association of pioglitazone use and bladder cancer through drug adverse event reporting. *Diabetes Care.* 2011;34:1369-1371.

76 Food and Drug Administration. FDA Drug Safety Communication. "Update to ongoing safety review of Actos (pioglitazone) and increased risk of bladder cancer." FDA Website. www.fda.gov/Drugs/DrugSafety/ucm259150.htm. Accessed September 5, 2012.

77 Agence Francaise de Securite Sanitaire des Produits de Sante (AFSSAPS). "Use of medications containing pioglitazone (Actos®, Competact®) suspended." June 9th, 2011. AFSSAPS website. www.afssaps.fr/var/afssaps_site/storage/original/application/4e293bcd0814c025b94d46d75 02a0958.pdf. Accessed September 5, 2012.

78 Bundesinstitut für Arzneimittel und Medizinprodukte (BfArM). "Pioglitazon - Europäische Arzneimittelagentur empfiehlt neue Kontraindikationen und Warnhinweise für pioglitazonhaltige Arzneimittel aufgrund eines leicht erhöhten Blasenkrebsrisikos [Pioglitazone: The European Medicines Agency recommends new contraindications and warnings for medicinal products containing pioglitazone due to a slightly increased risk of bladder cancer]." July 22, 2011. BfArM Website. www.bfarm.de/DE/Pharmakovigilanz/ risikoinfo/2011/pioglitazon.html?nn=1016416. Accessed September 5, 2012.

79 Lewis JD, Ferrara A, Peng T et al. Risk of bladder cancer among diabetic patients treated with pioglitazone: interim report of a longitudinal cohort study. *Diabetes Care.* 2011;34:916-922.

80 European Medicines Agency. European Medicines Agency recommends new contra-indications and warnings for pioglitazone to reduce small increased risk of bladder cancer. EMA website. www.ema.europa.eu/docs/en_GB/document_library/Press_release/2011/07/ WC500109176.pdf. Accessed September 5, 2012.

81 European Medicines Agency. "European Medicines Agency clarifies opinion on pioglitazone and the risk of bladder cancer. Positive benefit-risk balance confirmed as second and third line treatment." EMA Website. October 21, 2011. www.ema.europa.eu/docs/en_GB/document_ library/Press_release/2011/10/WC500116936.pdf. Accessed September 5, 2012.

Chapter 5

New and future therapies

Santosh Shankarnarayan and Gayatri Sreemantula

The available treatments for diabetes all have limitations, either because of side effects (particularly weight gain and hypoglycemia) or due to contraindications; hence there has been an increased emphasis on the development of newer and more effective agents for lowering glucose. Therapeutic challenges are encountered not only in achieving near-normal metabolic control, but also long-term maintenance, which remains notoriously difficult. It is also important to note that none of the current treatments used to treat diabetes has disease-modifying properties. However, over the past few years, several new antidiabetic agents acting on novel pathways have been developed, providing clinicians with more options for improving glycemic control and achieving recommended treatment targets. Some of the newly developed antidiabetic treatments are discussed in this chapter.

Inhaled insulins

Insulin is one of the most effective treatments available to lower glucose levels. However, it is associated with side effects such as hypoglycemia and weight gain and the fact that it has only been available in an injectable form has deterred some patients from starting insulin, despite its efficacy. In August 2006, Exubera was launched as the first inhaled insulin. However, amidst controversies surrounding the long-term safety of inhaled insulins and poor acceptance by patients and physicians, Exubera was withdrawn from the market in October 2007.

J. Vora and M. Evans (eds.), *Managing Diabetes*,
DOI: 10.1007/978-1-908517-81-4_5, © Springer Healthcare 2012

A new discrete insulin inhalation system, Technosphere, has since been developed, which uses a dry powder insulin formulation. The technosphere insulin (TI) is prepared by precipitating monomeric insulin from solution on to technosphere particles, which are comprised of a novel excipient, fumaryl diketopiperazine. The TI molecules have a uniform size and are further optimized for inhalation into the deep lung. The inhaler itself does not require manual activation or timing as it is triggered by patient inhalation. The unique pharmokokinetic properties of the TI facilitate peak insulin concentrations to be reached in 12 to 14 minutes following inhalation [1].

A recently published open-label randomized trial [2] compared prandial use of inhaled insulin plus basal insulin glargine to twice-daily biaspart insulin in patients with type 2 diabetes. After a 1-year follow-up period, similar reductions in glycated hemoglobin (HbA1c) were seen in both groups and the difference was 0.07% (standard error=0.102; 95% confidence interval [CI], 0.13–0.27). Patients on both inhaled insulin and insulin glargine had significantly lower weight gain and fewer hypoglycemic events. However, increased occurrence of cough and changes in pulmonary function were noted in the group receiving inhaled insulin plus insulin glargine. The cough abated with continued use and the changes in the pulmonary function tests were small and clinically insignificant.

More recently, further developments in inhaler technology have been subject to delays. Although there are Phase III trials supporting the application used in the MedTone delivery device, the manufacturer has opted to commercialize the next generation DreamBoat device. In 2011, the FDA issued a complete response letter requiring two clinical studies to be performed, one of which should have a head-to-head data comparison arm with the first generation MedTone inhaler [3]. These trials (Study 171 and Study 174) are currently in progress.

Thus, inhaled insulin offers an effective alternative to the conventional insulins and can help obtain better glycemic control with lower risk of weight gain and hypoglycemia. However, long-term safety data are still not available and further trials are required.

Oral hypoglycemic agents

Sodium-glucose transporter 2 inhibitors

As early as the second century, Aretaeus of Cappadocia, a Greek physician, recognized polyuria in patients with diabetes as a compensatory mechanism and concluded that the disorder was a fault of the kidneys. However, in more recent times the ability of the kidneys to influence glucose homeostasis has received little attention. In healthy people, the kidneys reabsorb nearly all of the filtered glucose (up to 180 mg in 24 hours) via the sodium-glucose transporter 2 (SGLT2), which is expressed in the proximal tubules. Patients with familial renal glycosuria, which is caused by mutation of the SLC5A2 gene that encodes SGLT2, remain asymptomatic without relevant loss of electrolytes and have no increase in the incidence of urogenital infections. Targeting this novel mechanism of glucose regulation via the kidneys has lead to the development of a new class of drugs: the SGLT2 inhibitors.

Dapagliflozin is a highly selective SGLT2 inhibitor, that can increase the urinary glucose excretion to between 45 and 80 g/day, resulting in improved glucose tolerance. A recent trial [4] investigating its efficacy as an add-on to metformin in patients with type 2 diabetes has shown a dose dependent reduction in HbA1c (0.84% reduction of HbA1c compared to 0.3% in the placebo group) (Figure 5.1) with low risk of hypoglycemia. Additionally in patients with type 2 diabetes inadequately controlled with metformin monotherapy, dapagliflozin as an add-on therapy was found to produce greater mean weight loss versus weight gain (1.2 kg; $P=0.0001$) when compared with an add-on sulfonylurea (eg, glipizide), as well as significantly increasing the proportion of patients achieving 5% body weight reduction and decreasing levels of hypoglycemia [5,6]. A reduction in body weight ($\geq 5\%$; Figure 5.2) and in both systolic and diastolic blood pressures was noted in all dapagliflozin-treated groups.

In some of the earlier trials, an increase in the risk for urinary tract infections had been noted [5,6]. By contrast, one recent trial showed no increase in the risk for urinary tract infections but a slight increase in genital infections [7]. In the presence of increased glucosuria, anomalies in the immune response and impaired cellular defence seen in diabetic

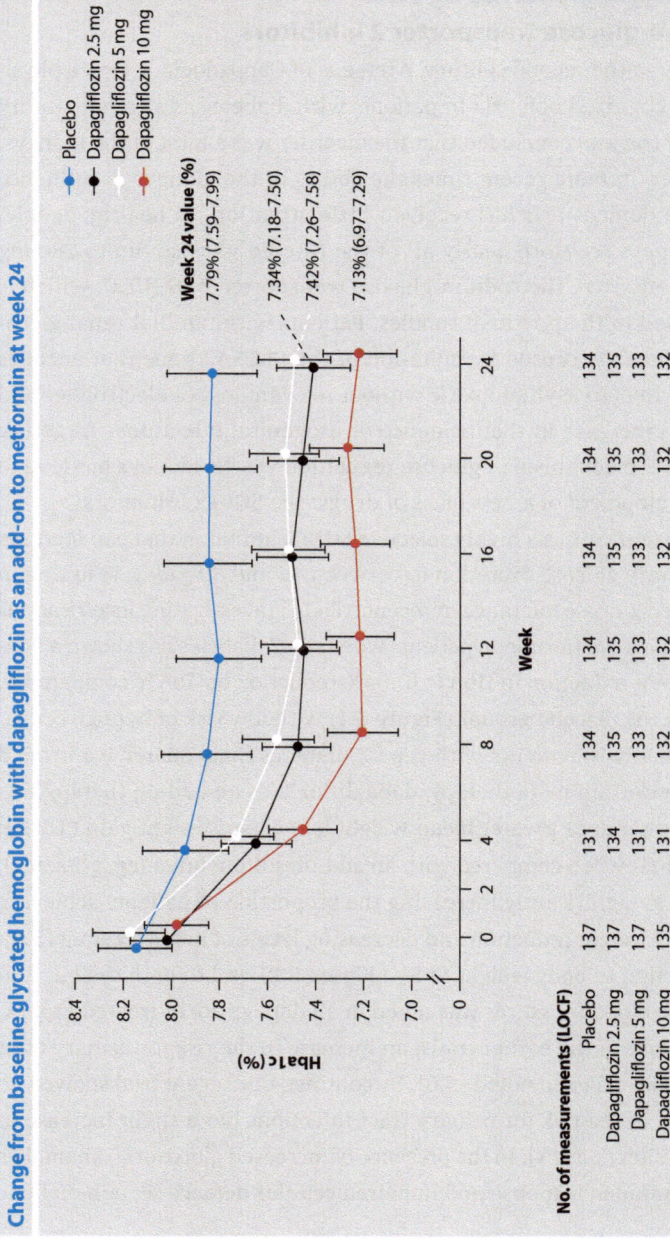

Figure 5.1 Change from baseline glycated hemoglobin with dapagliflozin as an add-on to metformin at week 24. HbA1c, glycated hemoglobin; LOCF, last observation carried forward. Reproduced with permission from Bailey et al [4].

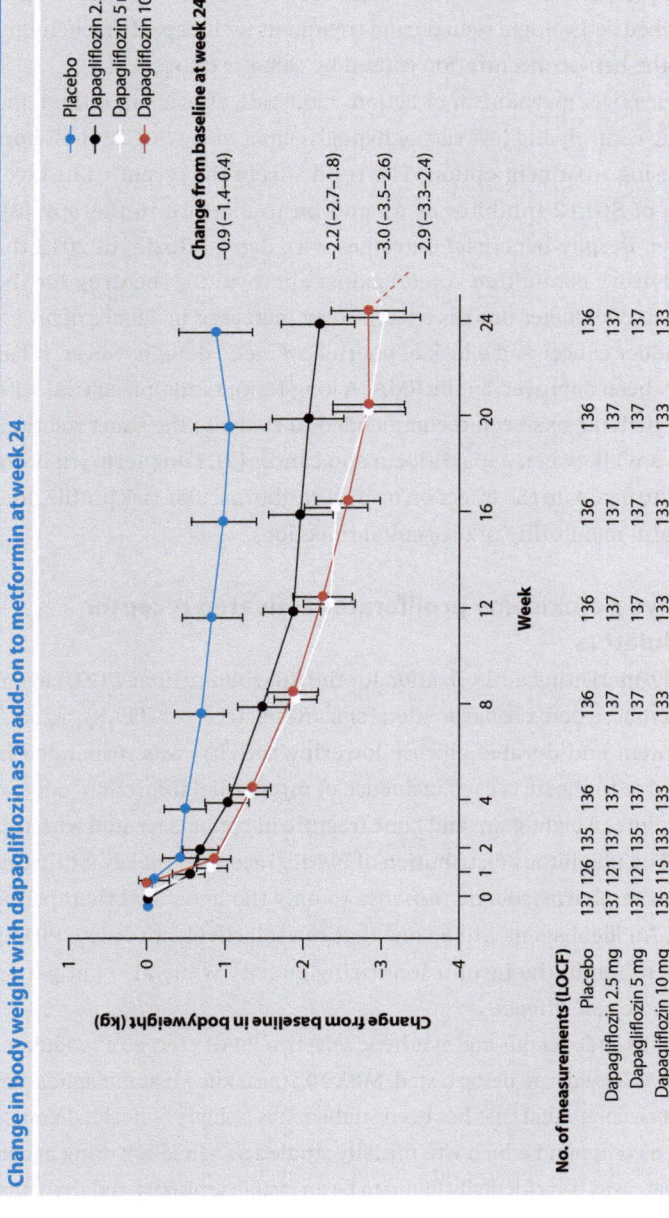

Figure 5.2 Change in body weight with dapagliflozin as an add-on to metformin at week 24. HbA1c, glycated hemoglobin; LOCF, last observation carried forward. Reproduced with permission from Bailey et al [4].

patients might be responsible for activation of any latent infection, such as asymptomatic bacteriuria. The increase in the blood urea nitrogen and packed cell volume seen during treatment with dapagliflozin might reflect the hemoconcentration caused by osmotic diuresis.

Their novel mechanism of action, moderate efficacy in optimizing glycemic control, and low risk of hypoglycemia make SGLT2 inhibitors a promising treatment option. The results from the recent trials favor the use of SGLT2 inhibitor as an add-on to metformin therapy [8]. However, despite beneficial outcomes with dapagliflozin, in 2012 the FDA advisory committee voted against approval for the drug for the treatment of diabetes due to concerns over increased incidence of breast and bladder cancer and a lack of pharmacokinetic data; however, it has recently been approved by the EMA. A long-term, randomized trial with 30,000 patients has been recommended to evaluate the exact relationship (if any) between dapagliflozin and cancer [9]. Long-term trials are needed to evaluate the effect on overall cardiovascular risk profile, and for careful monitoring of urogenital infections.

Selective peroxisome proliferator activated receptor γ modulators

Recently, marketing authorization for the thiazolidinedone (TZD) agent rosiglitazone, a peroxisome proliferator activated receptor (PPAR)γ agonist with potent and durable glucose lowering activity, was suspended in Europe due to the increased incidence of myocardial infarction, edema, heart failure, weight gain, and bone fracture in patients treated with this agent. The ubiquitous distribution of PPARγ receptors makes it difficult to limit the pharmacologic response to only the beneficial therapeutic effects. An ideal agent will be one that can selectively modulate PPARγ activity to retain the insulin-sensitizing activity while also mitigating unwelcome side effects.

Various endogenous and synthetic selective PPARγ receptor modulator (SPPARM) ligands are being tested. MBX-102 (also known as metaglidasen) is one such compound that has been studied. It is a single optical halofenate isomer, a compound which was initially studied as a lipid-lowering agent. Halofenate was coincidentally found to be an insulin sensitizer and the active optical isomer was developed as MBX-102. In diabetic rat models, MBX-102 showed glucose lowering properties and had insulin sensitizing effects (but with a much lower potency than rosiglitazone), without the weight gain seen with TZDs [10]. A more potent follow-on compound, MBX-2044, has now been developed and has completed Phase II clinical trials.

INT131 (also known as T131 and AMG131) is a synthetic non-TZD PPAR ligand designed to be a selective PPARγ modulator. In animal studies, INT131 showed similar or better efficacy and potency that is comparable with rosiglitazone (Figure 5.3) [11]. No significant weight gain, fatty replacement of the marrow, fluid retention, edema, cardiac hypertrophy or other signs of congestive heart failure was observed even after 6 months of treatment at exposures of more than 200 times greater than clinically efficacious concentrations [11]. INT 131 has completed Phase II development and is moving into Phase III clinical trials (a 24 week double-blind, placebo-controlled, active comparator [pioglitazone 45 mg] trial recruiting patients with poorly controlled type 2 diabetes currently being treated with sulfonylurea or sulphonylurea with metformin).

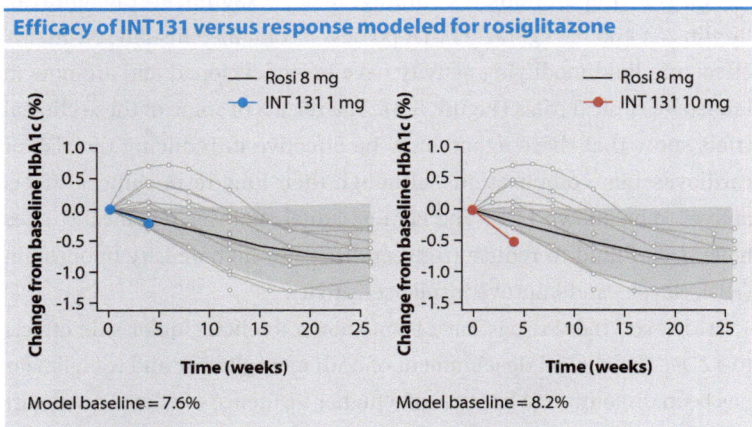

Efficacy of INT131 versus response modeled for rosiglitazone

Model baseline = 7.6%   Model baseline = 8.2%

Figure 5.3 Efficacy of INT131 versus response modeled for rosiglitazone. INT131 provided equal or greater glycemic efficacy compared with that predicted for maximal-dose thiazolidinedione. Results from a 4-week, Phase IIa, randomized, placebo-controlled study of patients with type 2 diabetes mellitus taking 1 or 10 mg INT131 as monotherapy (study INT131-T004) are compared with the response modeled for the same patient population taking a maximal dose (8 mg) of rosiglitazone (Rosi). In the absence of a direct comparison of INT131 to a thiazolidinedione, a meta-analysis approach provides quantitative comparative information. Reproduced with permission from INT131-004 Study Group [11].

Dual peroxisome proliferator activated receptor agonists (α and γ)

An antidiabetic drug that has the ability to optimize cardiovascular risk profiles and thereby lower mortality in patients with diabetes is very desirable. PPAR agonists have been thought to possess such properties. The PPARs are ligand-activated transcription factors of a nuclear hormone receptor superfamily comprising three subtypes: PPARα, PPARγ, and PPARδ/β. TZDs that activate PPARγ improve glycemic control by increasing peripheral insulin sensitivity and reducing hepatic glucose production, thereby helping to preserve beta cell function. The TZDs also have a modest beneficial effect of improving lipid profiles. Fibrates, on the other hand, through their interactions with PPARα receptors, mediate significant improvements in the atherogenic dyslipidemia but do not affect glycemic control. Hence, it can be postulated that a compound that can target both the α and γ receptors would provide the benefits of both TZDs and fibrates combined. The quest for such agents has led to the development of the 'glitazar' group of drugs.

Various preparations (eg, muraglitazar, tesaglitazar, ragaglitazar, farglitazar, and naveglitazar) that possess a combined insulin sensitizing effect and lipid modifying activity have been developed and are now in late-stage clinical trials (Figure 5.4). The results of some of these clinical trials show that these agents may be effective in reducing the risk of cardiovascular complications, although their long-term clinical effects are yet to be known [12]. The PPARα/γ dual agonists in clinical studies have been found to reduce triglycerides, raise high-density lipoprotein (HDL) levels, and improve insulin sensitivity.

However, these drugs have been shown to elicit similar side effects to TZDs. The clinical development of both muraglitazar and tesaglitazar has been discontinued because of a higher incidence of edema and heart failure, and tesaglitazar has been associated with decreases in glomerular filtration rate and elevations in serum creatinine. Muraglitazar has high affinity towards PPARγ and tesaglitazar has a preferential activity on the PPARα receptors. This lack of balance in binding affinity may lead to supratherapeutic activation of PPARα and γ receptors, which may be associated with adverse effects. Overexpression of the transcription factor

The synergistic beneficial actions of balanced PPARα/γ dual agonists

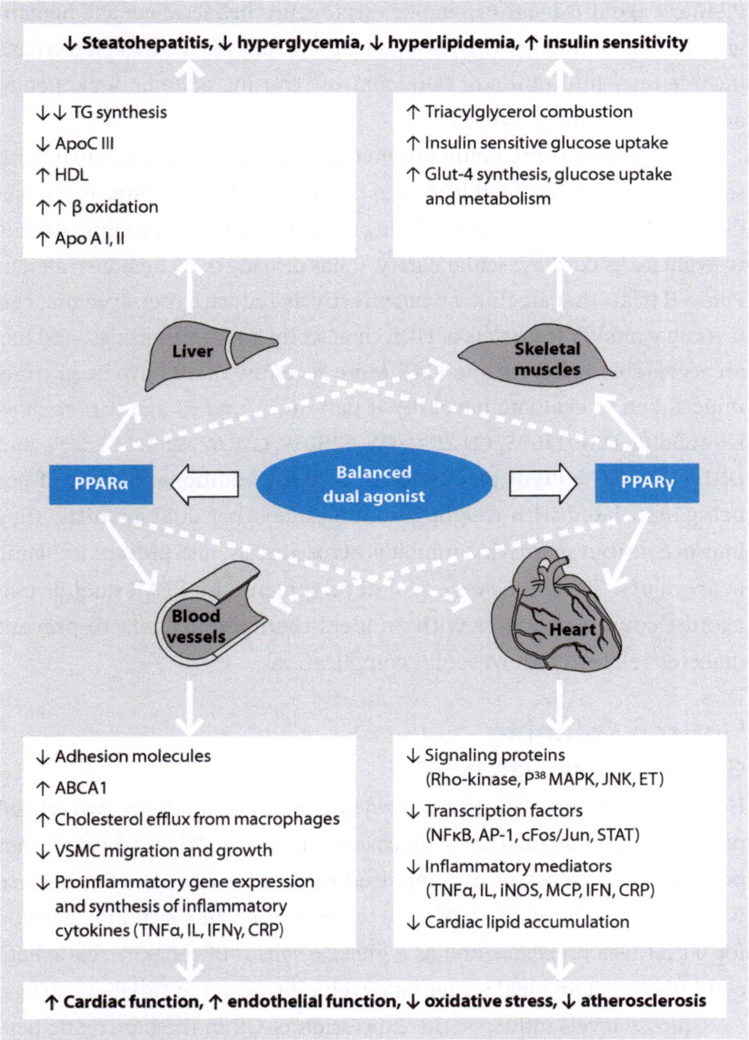

Figure 5.4 The synergistic beneficial actions of balanced PPARα/γ dual agonists.
ABCA1, adenosine triphosphate-binding cassette 1; AP-1, activator protein 1; Apo, apolipoprotein; CRP, C-reactive protein; ET, endothelin; FN, fibronectin; Glut-4, glucose transporter type 4; IFN, interferon; IL, interleukin; iNOS, inducible nitric oxide synthase; MAPK, mitogen-activated protein kinase; MCF, methylene chloride function; NFκB, nuclear factor kappa B; PPAR, peroxisome proliferator-activated receptor; STAT, signal transducers and activators of transcription; TG, triglyceride; TNF, tumor necrosis factor; VSMC, vascular smooth muscle cell.

early growth response-1 has been proposed to be a mechanism by which PPARα/γ agonists incite carcinogenesis (eg, urothelial cancer and hemangiosarcoma in rodents with ragaglitazar and MK 767). Other side effects include fatty infiltration of bone marrow causing anemia, leukopenia, and raised hepatic enzymes.

Current efforts are being targeted at developing dual agonists with selective and balanced PPARα/γ agonist activity [13]. Aleglitazar, a novel dual PPAR agonist, is currently being studied in large-scale clinical trials to evaluate its cardiovascular safety. It has already been demonstrated in Phase II trials that aleglitazar can effectively reduce hyperglycemia, can favorably modify the levels of HDL cholesterol and triglycerides, and has an acceptable safety profile [14]. More recently, there have been trials undertaken to evaluate novel PPAR pan- (α, γ, and δ) agonists such as LY-465608, DRF-11605, CS-204, GW-625019, GW 677954, PLX 204, and DRL-11605. The PPAR pan-agonists have the additional benefit of not being associated with weight gain, and like other dual agonists, they improve insulin sensitivity, inhibit atherosclerosis, and prevent ischemic heart injury. Thus, the successful development of a PPAR dual or pan agonist could provide us with an ideal therapeutic agent to prevent diabetes-related cardiovascular complications.

Horizon scanning
Glucokinase activators
Hepatic glucose uptake and glycogen synthesis clearance are two crucial processes in the regulation of glucose homeostasis. It is established that both of these processes are impaired in type 2 diabetes. Glucokinase (GK; also called hexokinase IV or D) serves as the rate-controlling enzyme for both these processes and as a glucose sensor of the pancreatic beta cells, making it an ideal target for developing newer antidiabetic drugs.

Glucose levels influence the expression of GK in the pancreatic beta cells in a concentration-dependent manner. High glucose levels can increase GK expression by up to 10 times, which enhances the biosynthesis and the release of insulin. Hepatic GK regulates energy homeostasis by playing a very important role in glycogen metabolism, glycolysis, the pentose-phosphate shunt, glucose oxidation, and associated oxidative phosphorylation and adenosine triphosphate production. GK also influences hepatic lipid metabolism and gluconeogenesis.

In type 2 diabetes, there appears to be a reduction in total GK that correlates with the reduced beta cell mass and function [15]. There also appears to be a right shift and blunting of the dose-dependency curve of glucose-stimulated insulin release. It is speculated that the constitutive expression of GK might be unaltered in the disease. There are several GK activators that are currently in clinical development. Some of these have also shown promising preclinical data and have advanced on to human clinical trials.

Glucagon receptor antagonists

Glucagon is produced by pancreatic alpha cells in the pancreas and, through hepatic gluconeogenesis, is responsible for postprandial hyperglycemia. In diabetic animal models, glucagon receptor antagonists or immunoneutralization of glucagon have been shown to improve glycemic control [16]. A number of glucagon receptor antagonists have been identified and are now in varying stages of clinical trials. These agents may provide a further alternative for optimizing postprandial hyperglycemia.

Sirtuins

In 1914, a young Professor F Peyton Rous described the beneficial effects on rats of a calorie-restricted diet. Over time, the molecular basis of caloric restriction was attributed to a family of nicotine adenine dinucleotide (NAD+)-dependent enzymes, now collectively termed sirtuins. To date, seven different members have been identified in the sirtuin family (SIRT 1–7), of which SIRT1 is the best studied. There is increasing interest in targeting this group of proteins because of the potential to treat diseases of aging such as type 2 diabetes, mitochondrial disorders, inflammation, cancer, and heart disease.

The diverse physiological roles of sirtuins have now been investigated in a number of animal trials (Figure 5.5). Sirtuins are thought to play a fundamental role in glucose homeostasis, and SIRT1-dependent deacetylation of peroxisome proliferator-activated receptor gamma coactivator-1α (PGC-1α) has been shown to regulate hepatic gluconeogenesis and fatty

The diverse physiological roles of the sirtuins

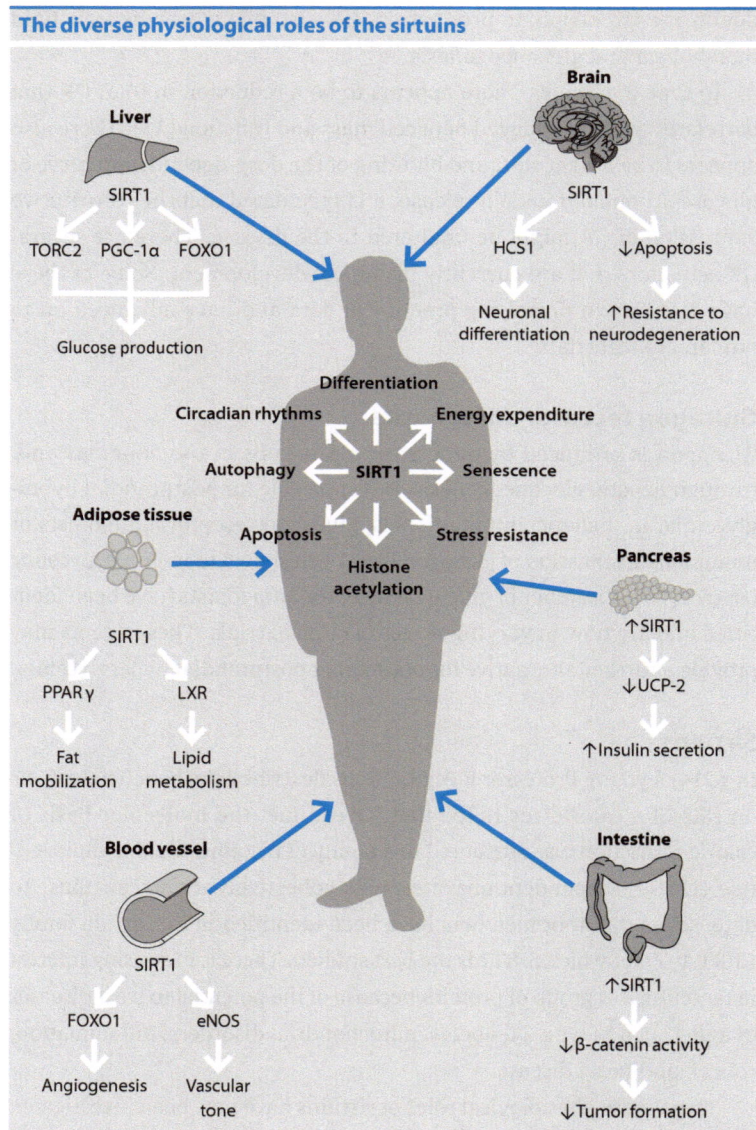

Figure 5.5 The diverse physiological roles of the sirtuins. eNOS, endothelial cell nitric oxide synthase; FOXO1, forkhead box protein 01; HCS1, hair cell soma A; LXR, liver X receptor; PGC-1α, peroxisome proliferator-activated receptor gamma [PPAR-γ] coactive 1-alpha; SIRT1, sirtuin 1; TORC2, transducer of regulated CAMP response element binding [CREB] protein 2; UCP-2, mitochondrial uncoupling protein 2.

acid oxidation in times of short- and long-term fasting [17]. In mice, sirtuins have been found to augment the glucose-stimulated insulin secretion and improve glucose tolerance [18]. Also, SIRT4 appears to be involved in regulating pancreatic insulin secretion through its interactions with the insulin degrading enzyme and the ADP-ribosylation of glutamate dehydrogenase (GDH) [19]. In animal models, treatment with resveratrol, a sirtuin activator found naturally in red wine, appears to protect against diet-induced obesity and glucose intolerance [18].

It has also been suggested that the sirtuins have a prominent role in aspects of age-dependent atherosclerosis. These effects may be related to the ability of SIRT1 to regulate lipid and cholesterol metabolism by modulating key nuclear receptors involved in reverse cholesterol transport. Recently, it has been observed that the SIRT1 might act as a non-traditional tumor suppressor; haploinsufficiency of SIRT1 in p53+/− mice resulted in increased tumor formation, while overexpressed SIRT1 reduced tumor formation [20].

The sirtuins bring with them a host of beneficial attributes. Our understanding has come from studies involving SIRT1 in animal models, but many questions remain unanswered. A better understanding of the other six mammalian sirtuins identified is required. Resveratrol and a few other newer agents with greater specificity have already entered human clinical trials. More studies are required to fully elucidate the roles of the sirtuins and to determine their disparate functions before pharmacological manipulation of sirtuin activity can become clinical practice.

Conclusions

Advances in our understanding of glucose homeostasis have helped in identifying novel drug targets for development of antidiabetic agents. These new agents can provide us with more options for achieving better glycemic control and overcoming treatment failure. Newer agents are geared to improve tolerability and safety and minimize side effects. It is to be hoped that the treatment of diabetes will be transformed with these distinctive agents, and that additional new therapies with disease-modifying properties will be developed, ultimately leading to a cure for diabetes in the future.

References

1   Pfützner A, Mann AE, Steiner SS. Technosphere/insulin: a new approach for effective delivery of human insulin via the pulmonary route. *Diabetes Techol Ther*. 2002;509-594.

2   Rosenstock J, Lorber DL, Gnudi L, et al. Prandial inhaled insulin plus basal insulin glargine versus twice-daily biaspart insulin for type 2 diabetes: a multicentre randomised trial. *Lancet*. 2010;375:2244-2253.

3   Kling J. Dreamboat sinks prospects for fast approval of inhaled insulin. *Nature Biotech*. 2011;29:175-176.

4   Bailey CJ, Gross LJ, Pieters A, et al. Effect of dapagliflozin in patients with type 2 diabetes who have inadequate glycemic control with metformin: a randomised, double-blind, placebo-controlled trial. *Lancet*. 2010;375:2223-2233.

5   Nauck MA, Del Prato S, Meier JJ, et al. Dapagliflozin versus glipizide as add-on therapy in patients with type 2 diabetes who have inadequate glycemic control with metformin: a randomized, 52-week, double-blind, active-controlled noninferiority trial. *Diabetes Care*. 2011;34:2015-2022.

6   Nauck M, Del Prato S, Rohwedder K, Theuerkauf A, Langkilde AM, Parikh S. Long-term efficacy and safety of add-on dapagliflozin vs add-on glipizide in patients with T2DM inadequately controlled with metformin: 2-year results. Poster presented at the 71st Scientific Sessions of the American Diabetes Association, June 24–28, 2011; San Diego, California.

7   Ferrannini E, Ramos SJ, Salsali A, Tang W, List JF. Dapagliflozin monotherapy in type 2 diabetic patients with inadequate glycemic control by diet and exercise: a randomized, double-blind, placebo-controlled, phase 3 trial. *Diabetes Care*. 2010;3322:2217-2224.

8   Aires I, Calado J. BI-10773, a sodium-glucose cotransporter 2 inhibitor for the potential oral treatment of type 2 diabetes mellitus. *Curr Opin Investig Drugs*. 2010;11:1182-1190.

9   Anderson SL, Marrs JC. Dapagliflozin for the treatment of type 2 diabetes. *Ann Pharmacother*. 2012;46:590-598.

10 Gregoire FM, Zhang F, Clarke HJ, et al. MBX-102/JNJ39659100, a novel peroxisome proliferator-activated receptor-ligand with weak transactivation activity retains antidiabetic properties in the absence of weight gain and edema. *Mol Endocrinol*. 2009;23:975-988.

11 INT131-004 Study Group. Selective modulation of PPARγ activity can lower plasma glucose without typical thiazolidinedione side-effects in patients with type 2 diabetes. *J Diabetes Complications*. 2011;25:151-158.

12 Higgins LS, DePaoli AM. Selective peroxisome proliferator-activated receptor γ (PPARγ) modulation as a strategy for safer therapeutic PPARg activation. *Am J Clin Nutr*. 2010;91(suppl):267S-272S.

13 Balakumar P, Rose M, Subrahmanya S, et al. PPAR dual agonists: Are they opening Pandora's box? *Pharmacological Res*. 2007;56:91-98.

14 Lecka-Czernik B. Aleglitazar, a dual PPARα and PPARγ agonist for the potential oral treatment of type 2 diabetes mellitus. *IDrugs*. 2010;11:793-807.

15 Matschinsky FM, Porte D Jr. Glucokinase activators (GKAs) promise a new pharmacotherapy for diabetics. *F1000 Med Rep*. 2010;2:43-48.

16 Sørensen H, Brand CL, Neschan S, et al. Immunoneutralization of endogenous glucagon reduces hepatic glucose output and improves long-term glycemic control in diabetic *ob/ob* mice. *Diabetes*. 2006;55:2843-2848.

17 Finkel T, Deng CX, Mostoslavsky R, et al. Recent progress in the biology and physiology of sirtuins. *Nature*. 2009;460:587-591.

18 Banks AS, Kon N, Knight C, et al. SirT1 gain of function increases energy efficiency and prevents diabetes in mice. *Cell Metab*. 2008;8:333-341.

19 Haigis MC, Mostoslavsky R, Haigis KM, et al. SIRT4 inhibits glutamate dehydrogenase and opposes the effects of calorie restriction in pancreatic beta cells. *Cell*. 2006;126:941-954.

20 Lim CS. SIRT1: tumor promoter or tumor suppressor? *Med Hypotheses*. 2006;67:341-344.

Chapter 6

Managing the complications of diabetes

Santosh Shankarnarayan

Chronic hyperglycemia is associated with many serious complications (eg, heart disease, stroke, end-stage renal disease [ESRD], nerve disease, dental disease, blindness, amputations) and premature mortality [1]. The results from the Diabetes Control and Complications Trial (DCCT) and the UK Prospective Diabetes Study (UKPDS) convincingly demonstrate the importance of good glycemic control to prevent microvascular complications of diabetes [2,3].

Pathogenesis

Hyperglycemia is considered to be one of the major factors involved in the development of complications in patients with diabetes. Various pathways have been recognized through which elevated blood sugar is thought to mediate cellular dysfunction and damage. Some of the better understood pathways attribute the cellular injury to the products of glucose metabolism (eg, sorbitol, N-acetyl-glucosamine, N-carboxymethyl-lysine, pentosidine, and methylglyoxal derivatives). Sorbitol is formed as a product of enzymatic breakdown of glucose by aldose reductase and is thought to trigger a variety of intracellular changes [4]. There is now a large body of evidence suggesting that advanced glycation end products are important pathogenetic mediators of almost all diabetic complications. In patients with poorly controlled diabetes, there is increased production of

J. Vora and M. Evans (eds.), *Managing Diabetes*,
DOI: 10.1007/978-1-908517-81-4_6, © Springer Healthcare 2012

advanced glycation endproducts (AGEs), which cause functional altera-tions of intracellular proteins and alter interactions with AGEs, matrix and other cells. Also, intermediates like N-acetyl-glucosamine formed during glucose metabolism in the hexosamine pathway accumulate in the presence of high glucose levels and cause a permanent modifica-tion of proteins and transcription factors. In addition, elevated glucose levels are responsible for the activation of the enzyme protein kinase C, which alters cell function [5]. Thus, poor glycemic control through various mechanisms exerts direct and indirect effects on the vascular tree, resulting in significant morbidity and mortality. In this chapter, the deleterious effects of uncontrolled hyperglycemia are discussed as microvascular (nephropathy, retinopathy and neuropathy) and macro-vascular complications (cardiovascular disease, cerebrovascular disease and peripheral vascular disease).

Microvascular complications of diabetes

Nearly half of people with type 2 diabetes show signs of microvascular complications at the time of diagnosis. The complications may begin 5 to 6 years before the diagnosis but the actual onset of diabetes may be 10 years or more before clinical diagnosis [6]. By contrast, in type 1 dia-betes, an increased incidence of microvascular complications is usually not observed until 10 years after the initial diagnosis.

Diabetic nephropathy

Diabetes is the single most common cause of ESRD and accounts for up to 40% of new cases of the condition. Almost one in three patients with type 2 diabetes develops overt kidney disease and patients with type 2 diabetes are commonly found to have albuminuria and overt nephropa-thy at the time, or soon after, of the diagnosis of diabetes [7]. Up to 50% of the patients with type 1 diabetes will develop ESRD within 10 years and 75% within 20 years [7]. Apart from poor glycemic control, factors such as cigarette smoking, hyperlipidemia, hypertension, genetics, and ethnicity have been found to affect the progression of nephropathy [7].

All patients with type 2 diabetes should be screened for microalbu-minuria at diagnosis, while individuals with type 1 diabetes should be tested after 5 years of disease duration. In the absence of microalbuminuria on initial screening, the test should be performed annually. Albumin excretion is regarded as abnormal if urine levels are 30 mg/24 hour and defined as microalbuminuria for values up to 299 mg/24 hour, beyond which it is macroalbuminuria (>300 mg/24 hour) (Figure 6.1) [8].

The natural history of diabetic nephropathy has been better defined in type 1 diabetes than type 2 diabetes. Mogenson has described five distinct stages of diabetic nephropathy [9]. These include a stage of renal hypertrophy with hyperfiltration and normal renal function. This is followed by a silent phase with early histological changes without clinically evident renal disease; the progression of histological changes leads to the development of microalbuminuria and is described as incipient diabetic nephropathy. This stage is invariably followed by established or overt diabetic nephropathy. There is relentless decline in the renal function during this stage accompanied by increasing proteinuria. Without intervention ESRD ensues following a median of 7 years of persistent proteinuria and requires dialysis [9].

The DCCT study showed previous intensive treatment resulting in near normal glycemia had an extended benefit in delaying the onset and progression of diabetic nephropathy [4]. However, intensive glycemic control may not slow the rate of progressive renal injury in patients once overt proteinuria (macroalbuminuria) has developed [10,11]. At this late stage, there is often marked glomerulosclerosis. Only antihypertensive therapy (preferably with angiotensin-converting enzyme [ACE] inhibitors, and angiotensin receptor blockers) and dietary protein restriction have been shown to slow the rate of progressive disease or reverse established lesions [12]. With aggressive treatment of hypertension (Figure 6.2) and

Diagnostic limits for normo-, micro-, and macroalbuminuria		
	24 hour urine collection	First morning or spot urine sample
Normoalbuminuria	<30 mg/24 hour	<2.5 mg/mmol (for men)
		<3.5 mg/mmol (for women)
Microalbuminuria	30–300 mg/24 hour	2.5–30 mg/mmol (for men)
		3.5–30 mg/mmol (for women)
Macroalbuminuria	>300 mg/24 hour	>30 mg/mmol

Figure 6.1 Diagnostic limits for normo-, micro- ,and macroalbuminuria.

hyperlipidemia and improvement of glycemic control, the need for renal replacement therapy may be delayed for several years [13]. Renal physicians would like to see patients with diabetic nephropathy earlier and referral for renal replacement should be instigated when serum creatinine levels start to rise, and certainly before they reach 300 μmol/L. Renal transplantation offers the best method of treatment for suitable patients, while hemodialysis is indicated in patients unsuitable for transplantation.

The UKPDS demonstrated that there was an increasing trend towards cardiovascular mortality with worsening diabetic nephropathy ($P<0.0001$), with an annual rate of 12.1% for those with elevated plasma creatinine (≥ 175 mmol/L) or undergoing renal replacement therapy [4]. Most of the deaths were due to cardiovascular causes; the reasons are unclear but are thought to be related to the clustering of risk factors (hypertension, hyperlipidemia, smoking, and increased platelet/fibrinogen aggregability) in patients with renal dysfunction [13]. Survival rates for type 1 patients with overt diabetic nephropathy appear to be improving, and is now 80% (compared with 25% in the 1950s) [14]. Prevention of diabetic nephropathy and premature cardiovascular and renal deaths in patients with type 2 diabetes has improved over the last 20 years but still remains a major challenge for clinical medicine [15,16].

Diabetic retinopathy

Diabetic retinopathy is the leading cause of blindness among working age adults in developed countries [17]. The development of diabetic retinopathy is related to both the severity of diabetes and hypertension. It is now evident that most patients with type 1 diabetes develop diabetic retinopathy within 20 years of diagnosis [18], and as early as 7 years before the diagnosis of diabetes in patients with type 2 diabetes [19]. The prevalence of retinopathy increases with the duration of diabetes.

Microangiopathy and capillary occlusion are central to the development of diabetic retinopathy [20]. Accumulation of increasing amounts of sorbitol, AGEs, and oxidative free radicals in the cells have all been linked to the formation of microaneurysm, thickening of basement membranes, and loss of pericytes. Increasing levels of vascular endothelial growth factor (VEGF) and transforming growth factor beta in response

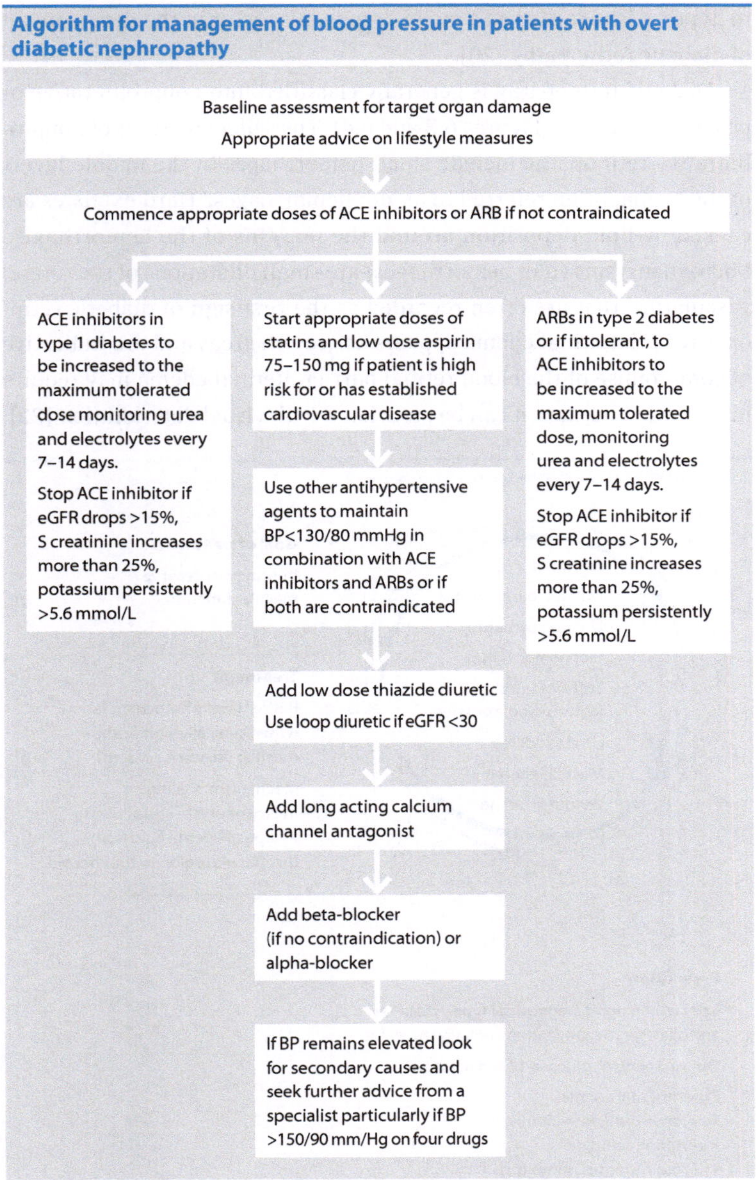

Algorithm for management of blood pressure in patients with overt diabetic nephropathy

Baseline assessment for target organ damage

Appropriate advice on lifestyle measures

Commence appropriate doses of ACE inhibitors or ARB if not contraindicated

ACE inhibitors in type 1 diabetes to be increased to the maximum tolerated dose monitoring urea and electrolytes every 7–14 days.

Stop ACE inhibitor if eGFR drops >15%, S creatinine increases more than 25%, potassium persistently >5.6 mmol/L

Start appropriate doses of statins and low dose aspirin 75–150 mg if patient is high risk for or has established cardiovascular disease

Use other antihypertensive agents to maintain BP<130/80 mmHg in combination with ACE inhibitors and ARBs or if both are contraindicated

ARBs in type 2 diabetes or if intolerant, to ACE inhibitors to be increased to the maximum tolerated dose, monitoring urea and electrolytes every 7–14 days.

Stop ACE inhibitor if eGFR drops >15%, S creatinine increases more than 25%, potassium persistently >5.6 mmol/L

Add low dose thiazide diuretic

Use loop diuretic if eGFR <30

Add long acting calcium channel antagonist

Add beta-blocker (if no contraindication) or alpha-blocker

If BP remains elevated look for secondary causes and seek further advice from a specialist particularly if BP >150/90 mm/Hg on four drugs

Figure 6.2 Algorithm for management of blood pressure in patients with overt diabetic nephropathy. ACE, angiotensin converting enzyme; ARB, angiotensin II receptor blocker; P, blood pressure. eGFR, estimated glomerular filtration rate. Reproduced with permission from Breyer [13].

to hypoxia is regarded as a major angiogenic factor in the development of diabetic retinopathy [20].

Diabetic retinopathy is generally classified into nonproliferative or proliferative forms (Figures 6.3 and 6.4). The salient features of nonproliferative retinopathy include small hemorrhages in the middle layers of the retina, often referred to as 'dot hemorrhages.' Hard exudates are caused by lipid deposition around the margins of the hemorrhages. Microaneurysms (blot hemorrhages) are small dilatations of the retinal vasculature that are often regarded as the first sign of diabetic retinopathy [21]. Retinal edema appears as greyish areas and are indicative of compromise of the blood retinal barrier. Retinal edema may require intervention because it can be associated with visual deterioration [22].

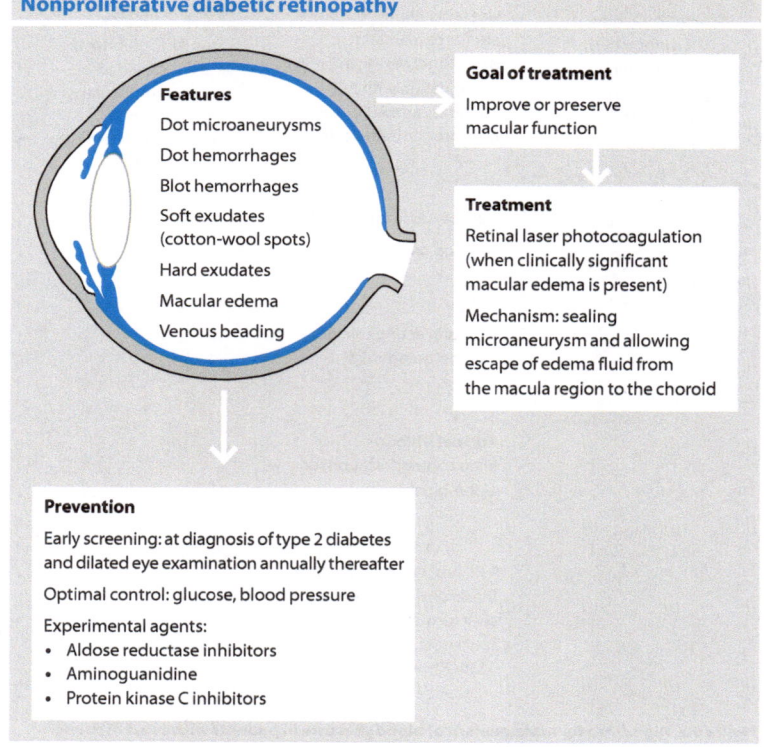

Figure 6.3 Nonproliferative diabetic retinopathy. Reproduced with permission from Sunder et al [22].

Proliferative diabetic retinopathy is characterized by formation of new blood vessels on the surface of the retina and can be complicated by vitreous hemorrhage. White areas on the retina (so-called, 'cotton wool spots'), can be a sign of impending proliferative retinopathy. Tractional retinal detachment from a vitreous hemorrhage can lead to blindness. Laser photocoagulation can prevent proliferative retinopathy and blindness.

Diabetic maculopathy is another important cause of visual loss in type 2 diabetes and may be exudative, edematous, or ischemic. In general, maculopathy is a progressive condition and good control of blood sugars and blood pressure can prevent or delay it. Laser photocoagulation is the only definitive treatment that is helpful to limit further damage and preserve the visual acuity.

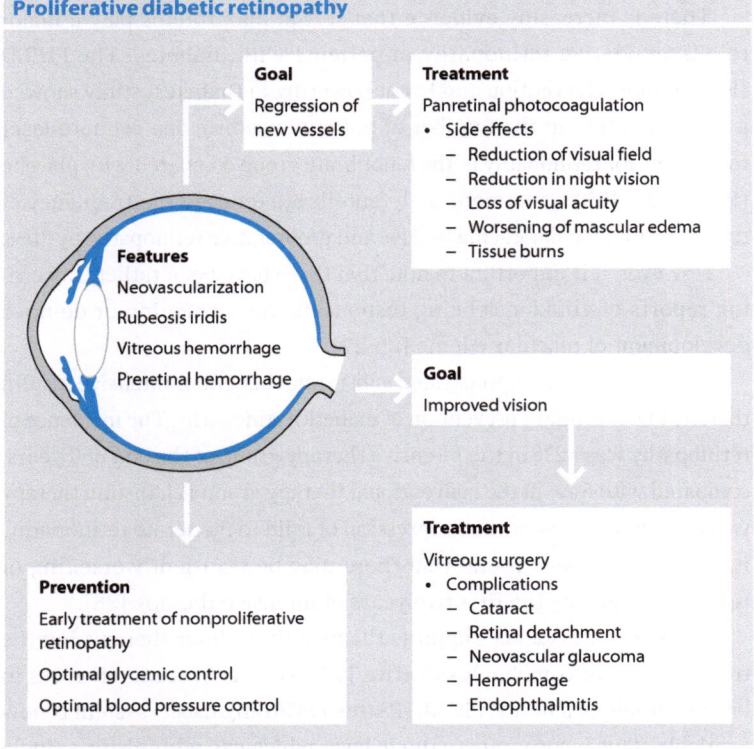

Proliferative diabetic retinopathy

Goal
Regression of new vessels

Treatment
Panretinal photocoagulation
• Side effects
  – Reduction of visual field
  – Reduction in night vision
  – Loss of visual acuity
  – Worsening of mascular edema
  – Tissue burns

Features
Neovascularization
Rubeosis iridis
Vitreous hemorrhage
Preretinal hemorrhage

Goal
Improved vision

Treatment
Vitreous surgery
• Complications
  – Cataract
  – Retinal detachment
  – Neovascular glaucoma
  – Hemorrhage
  – Endophthalmitis

Prevention
Early treatment of nonproliferative retinopathy
Optimal glycemic control
Optimal blood pressure control

Figure 6.4 Proliferative diabetic retinopathy. Reproduced with permission from Sunder et al [22].

Therefore close surveillance for the existence or progression of retinopathy in patients with diabetes are key priorities for reducing the morbidity of diabetic eye disease [22,23]. If left untreated, diabetic retinopathy will have a serious effect on the patient's eye sight.

Multiple risk factor treatment is beneficial for reducing diabetic retinopathy endpoints. The Steno-2 trial provided evidence that an average of 13.3 years of intensified management, which comprised achieving targets of glycated hemoglobin (HbA1c) <6.5%, fasting cholesterol <4.5 mmol/L, triglycerides <1.7 mmol/L, systolic blood pressure <130 mmHg, and treatment with renin-angiotensin blockers, statins, and a low-dose aspirin, resulted in a significant reduction in the progression of diabetic retinopathy of 43% ($P=0.02$) and a significant reduction of blindness ($P=0.03$) [24].

There is increasing evidence that serum lipoproteins play a major role in exudative retinopathy in patients with diabetes. The FIELD (Fenofibrate Intervention and Event Lowering in Diabetes) study showed a 30% reduction in the number of patients needing one or more laser treatments for retinopathy in the fenofibrate group compared with placebo ($P<0.0003$) [25]. Treatment with fenofibrate reduced the frequency of treatment for macular edema by 31% and proliferative retinopathy by 30%.

However, it is important to note that there have been rather concerning reports of glitazones being responsible for worsening or de novo development of macular edema [26,27].

The DCCT study demonstrated substantial benefit of intensive insulin therapy in the primary prevention of diabetic retinopathy. The incidence of retinopathy was 12% in the intensive therapy group at the end of 9 years, compared with 54% in the conventional therapy group [2]. Insulin therapy was also shown to slow the progression of mild to moderate retinopathy. It has however been found that there may be transient worsening of retinopathy during the first two years of intensive therapy [28].

The current evidence supports the benefits of laser therapy, but the treatment is not completely effective [29]. With the recent advances in laser technology a new PASCAL (PAttern SCAning Laser) system is now available. This incorporates a diode laser which can administer a single spot or a predetermined grid of laser burns with the single depression of the laser foot pedal, making it more effective with less discomfort [30,31].

Evaluations of AGE inhibitors in the treatment of diabetic retinopathy are underway [19]. Treatments with antioxidants such as vitamin E may attenuate some vascular dysfunction but have yet to be shown to alter the development or progression of retinopathy [19,32]. More recently, large randomized trials of intravitreal injection of VEGF inhibitors, such as pegaptanib for the treatment of diabetic retinopathy, are underway. Among the other newer therapies available is ruboxistaurin, which blocks the protein kinase C pathway. These newer therapies have shown a reduction in the need for laser treatment and minimizes visual loss in patients with diabetic maculopathy [33].

In the UK, there is now a comprehensive diabetes retinopathy screening service which enables an accurate retinopathy status to be known for most patients with diabetes. The results of the retinal screening are made available to those receiving diabetes care.

Diabetic neuropathy

Diabetic neuropathy is the most common form of neuropathy in the western world. Approximately 50% of patients with diabetes have mild-to-severe forms of neuropathy [34]. Several distinct forms of neuropathy are associated with diabetes; the most frequently encountered forms are summarized in Figure 6.5.

The most common form of diabetic neuropathy is the distal symmetric sensorimotor neuropathy, which occurs in a glove and stocking pattern (characterized by symptoms like burning, shooting pain, tingling

---

Diabetic neuropathy

- Distal symmetric sensorimotor neuropathy
- Focal mononeuropathies:
  - Cranial mononeuropathy (especially cranial nerves III, VI, and IV)
  - Peripheral mononeuropathy (especially median and peroneal nerves)
  - Mononeuropathy multiplex
- Autonomic neuropathy
- Polyradiculopathies:
  - Diabetic amyotrophy (lumbar polyradiculopathy)
  - Thoracic polyradiculopathy

Figure 6.5 Diabetic neuropathy.

sensations and allodynia). Diabetic peripheral neuropathy results in recurrent lower extremity infections and ulcerations, and is a major contributor to nontraumatic lower extremity amputations (more than 60% of cases) [35]. Diabetic mononeuropathies occur mainly in older patients and are more common in males. Third cranial nerve palsies are the most common, although other nerve lesions have also described. When two or more nerve palsies occur in a short timeframe, other causes of mononeuritis multiplex (eg, vasculitis) must be excluded. Proximal motor neuropathy is associated with weakness of the proximal muscles of both the lower limbs. It begins unilaterally but often spreads bilaterally. Slow, sometimes incomplete, recovery usually occurs and may take several months to a year (or longer).

Autonomic neuropathy is seen in diabetic patients, though the exact prevalence is unknown. There is a wide spectrum of autonomic symptoms, including orthostatic hypotension, diminished or absence of sweating in feet, gustatory sweating, gastroparesis, nocturnal diarrhea, sexual dysfunction (male impotence), bladder incontinence, cardiovascular damage, and loss of awareness of acute hypoglycemia. Many studies have suggested that once symptomatic autonomic neuropathy is present, the prognosis for the patient is poor [35].

There are three proposed stages of peripheral neuropathy: functional (reversible, with only biochemical alteration in nerve function); structural (may be reversible, associated with structural change in nerve fibers); and nerve death (irreversible, there is critical decrease in nerve fiber density and neuronal death) [36]. The best way to manage diabetic neuropathy is through primary prevention, management of early symptoms, and effective pain relief [37–39].

The main goals of treatment of diabetic neuropathy are: 1) to improve glycemic control and other risk factors of neuropathy; 2) to treat symptoms such as neuropathic pain; and 3) to prevent and manage complications such as foot ulcers, amputations, and gastroparesis. Various agents have been evaluated in clinical trials; some of the treatments currently licensed for use in diabetic neuropathy include tricyclic antidepressants (TCAs), anticonvulsants, opioids, and topical treatments such as capsaicin and lidocaine (Figure 6.6).

Medications used in the treatment of diabetic neuropathy

Medication class	No. of studies	Pooled odds ratio (95% CI) Efficacy*	Withdrawal
Antidepressants			
• Tricyclic antidepressants	3	22.24 (5.83–84.75)	2.32 (0.56–9.69)
• Citalopram	1	3.5 (0.3–38.2)	5.6 (0.3–38.2)
• Duloxetine 60 mg	2	2.55 (1.73–3.77)	2.36 (1.05–5.35)
• Duloxetine 120 mg	2	2.10 (1.03–4.27)	4.65 (2.18–9.94)
Anticonvulsants			
• Traditional[†]	3	5.33 (1.77–16.02)	1.51 (0.33–6.96)
• Newer generation[‡]	4	3.25 (2.27–4.66)	2.98 (1.75–5.07)
Opioids	3	4.25 (2.33–7.77)	4.06 (1.16–14.21)
Topical agents			
• Capsaicin	1	2.37 (1.32–4.26)	4.02 (1.45–11.16)

Figure 6.6 Medications used in the treatment of diabetic neuropathy. *Odds ratio for 50% or moderate reduction in pain compared to placebo. [†]Carbamazepine, sodium valproate. [‡]Gabapentin, pregabalin.

TCAs can be divided into two groups: tertiary amines, which block serotonin reuptake more than the norepinephrine reuptake, and secondary amines, which block norepinephrine reuptake more than the serotonin reuptake in the central nervous system [39]. Common side effects of TCAs include blurred vision, dry mouth, orthostatic hypotension, constipation and urinary retention. Secondary amines have fewer side effects and hence may be preferred over tertiary amines. Duloxetine is specifically approved for the management of pain associated with diabetic neuropathy and can be prescribed at a treatment dose of 60 mg once or twice daily.

Anticonvulsants such as carbamazepine, gabapentin, and pregabalin have been found to be effective in the treatment of painful neuropathies. They exert their effect by stabilizing the neurons through inhibition of ionic conductance. Carbamazepine is used at a dose of 100 mg once or twice daily (not to exceed 1,200 mg daily) to treat diabetic peripheral neuropathy. Adverse effects like dizziness, drowsiness, and lightheadness can be experienced transiently. At higher doses ataxia, diplopia, and nystagmus can occur.

Gabapentin and pregabalin are effective in the treatment of neuropathic pain. Meta-analyses of the two treatments showed that pregabalin has lower dosage needed to treat values for pain reduction compared with gabapentin, with a similar side effect profile [40]. Also pregabalin has a simple dosing and titration regimen compared with gabapentin. Initial doses of 150 mg/day of pregabalin can be used for treatment of both central and peripheral neuropathic pain.

Opioid analgesics have been used in the treatment of diabetic neuropathy albeit with variable efficacy and based on limited evidence. In a randomized control trial, oxcodone was evaluated as an initial therapy in 150 patients with moderate-to-severe pain due to diabetic neuropathy. In comparison to placebo, patients on oxycodone experienced only a slight improvement in the intensity of the pain [41]. The role of opioids may be limited due to the risk of physical dependance, tolerance, and adverse effects.

Tramadol is an opioid-like, centrally acting, synthetic non-narcotic analgesic that induces serotonin release, and inhibits the reuptake of norepinephrine. Randomized controlled trials have demonstrated a clinically and statistically significant reduction in pain intensity when patients were treated with tramadol [42].

Topical agents like capsaicin, a chilli pepper extract, are commonly used for local pain relief because they do not pose a risk for systemic toxicity. The analgesic effect is produced by depletion of substance P on the unmyelinated primary afferent nerve fibers. Patients should be advised that repeated use is necessary for pain relief and to wash hands thoroughly after each application.

The various manifestations of autonomic neuropathy can prove to be challenging to treat. Orthostatic hypotension may be treated with support stockings, salt tablets, or fludrocortisone. Gastroparesis can cause severe dehydration and metabolic imbalance. If this occurs, appropriate supportive therapy should be provided, and hospitalization for administration of intravenous fluids and correction of metabolic derangements may be required. Some patients with diabetic gastroparesis may benefit from metoclopramide or erythromycin. In severe cases, gastric pacing has been used.

Macrovascular complications of diabetes

Accelerated atherosclerosis of large and medium sized vessels is one of the hallmarks of diabetic macrovascular disease. Patients with diabetes are at increased risk of myocardial infarction, stroke, and lower-extremity gangrene [43]. The most effective approach for the prevention of macrovascular complications appears to be multifactorial risk-factor reduction (including glycemic control, smoking cessation, aggressive blood pressure control, and treatment of dyslipidemia).

Cardiovascular disease

People with diabetes are two to four times more likely to develop cardiovascular disease than those without diabetes [3]. Several risk factors contribute to the development of coronary heart disease, including poor glycemic control, hypertension, high cholesterol and lifestyle (diet, cigarette smoking, and lack of exercise). Mechanisms that contribute to the increased risk of coronary heart disease include endothelial dysfunction, hypercoagulability, impaired fibrinolysis, platelet aggregability, oxidative stress, sympathovagal imbalance, and glucose toxicity. Insulin resistance is associated with a significantly greater risk for the development of cardiovascular disease [3]. Insulin resistance creates a proinflammatory, prothrombotic environment and is associated with the development of other cardiovascular risk factors such as hypertension, atherogenic dyslipidemia, and microalbuminuria.

It was convincingly proven by the DCCT study [3] that a sustained period of glycemic control had a lasting benefit in reducing cardiovascular morbidity and mortality; the difference in the HbA1c levels between the intensive and conventional treatment groups at the end of the DCCT trial were 7.4 and 9.1%, respectively. Additionally, there was a 42% decrease in any cardiovascular event and a 57% reduction in a serious cardiovascular event (nonfatal myocardial infarction, stroke, or cardiovascular disease-related death; 95% CI, 12–79%) in the intensive therapy group when compared with the conventional treatment group of DCCT [3].

There is substantial evidence to demonstrate that lowering blood pressure can independently reduce cardiovascular events. The UKPDS data showed a linear relationship between the mean systolic blood pressure and cardiovascular disease, diabetes-related death, and all-cause mortality, with no apparent blood pressure threshold [4]. There was also a further accrual of cardiovascular risk with every increase in the systolic blood pressure from 120 mmHg onwards. In addition, tight blood pressure control was associated with significant reductions not only in microvascular endpoints but also for the risk of stroke (44%) and diabetes-related death (32%). The Action in Diabetes and Vascular disease: preterAx and dimicroN mr Controlled Evaluation (ADVANCE) trial reaffirmed the importance of blood pressure control in the reduction of cardiovascular events and also provided some data regarding the benefits of treating blood pressure among diabetic patients with prehypertension and even normotension [44]. While more evidence is required to revise the treatment targets for blood pressure, the current NICE guidelines (CG66) recommend a target blood pressure of 140/80 mmHg for diabetic patients with hypertension and a target blood pressure of <130/80 mmHg in patients with evidence of retinopathy, nephropathy, or evidence of cerebrovascular damage [45]. The seventh report of the Joint National Committee on prevention, detection, evaluation, and treatment of high blood pressure (JNC 7) recommends that diabetic patients maintain a blood pressure of <130/80 mmHg [46].

Strong evidence that lowering serum cholesterol decreases the risk of coronary heart disease comes from clinical trials of statin drugs. The Collaborative AtoRvastatin Diabetes Study (CARDS) and the Heart Protection Study (HPS) strongly suggest that all type 2 diabetic patients should receive statin therapy [47,48]. The pre-treatment low density lipoprotein (LDL) cholesterol level did not influence the decrease in the relative coronary heart disease risk. In the HPS study, there did not appear to be any threshold below which statin therapy was ineffective. The evidence from randomized statin trials that coronary heart disease risk reduction with statins is linearly related to the achieved decrease in LDL cholesterol supports the recommendation that therapeutic LDL cholesterol targets should be 2 mmol/L or less.

Cerebrovascular disease

Various cerebrovascular events can result from either inadequate blood flow to the brain (cerebral ischemia) or from hemorrhages into the parenchyma of the central nervous system. Patients with type 2 diabetes have a two-fold increased risk of stroke within the first five years of diagnosis, compared with the general population [49]. Patients with type 1 diabetes also bear a disproportionate burden of vascular disease. Observational studies have shown that the cerebrovascular mortality rate is high at all ages in patients with type 1 diabetes [50]. The risk of stroke-related dementia and recurrence, as well as stroke-related mortality, are elevated in patients with diabetes [51].

Acute treatments of ischemic stroke have been transformed over the recent years. Intravenous fibrinolytic therapy within three hours of the onset of stroke is now proven to be of substantial benefit. An evidence base of 21 completed randomized controlled clinical trials support this therapy. Two large trials involving approximately 40,000 patients indicated that the early use of aspirin in patients with acute ischemic stroke who were not treated with a fibrinolytic agent was associated with a small but significant reduction in mortality and stroke recurrence [52,53]. These studies in combination would suggest that for every 1000 stroke patients treated with aspirin, nine deaths or nonfatal recurrences would be prevented in the first few weeks, and approximately 13 fewer patients would be dead or dependent at 6 months. However, aspirin should not be given for the first 24 hours in patients receiving thrombolytic therapy, as it is associated with an increased risk of intracranial hemorrhage and death.

Peripheral vascular disease

The metabolic derangements associated with diabetes predispose patients to develop an atherosclerotic occlusive disease. Diabetic patients are at a three or four-fold higher risk of developing peripheral vascular disease (PVD) [54,55]. The age of the patient, duration of diabetes and presence of peripheral neuropathy, along with other factors (eg, hypertension, hyperlipidemia, cigarette smoking) increase the risk for developing PVD. Elevated levels of C-reactive protein, fibrinogen, homocysteine, apolipoprotein B, lipoprotein (A), and plasma viscosity are also potential risk factors for PVD. The two cardinal symptoms of PVD are intermittent claudication and pain at rest. Pain at rest is indicative of critical limb ischemia. PVD is a major risk factor for lower extremity amputations.

The Clopidogrel versus Aspirin in Patients at Risk of Ischaemic Events (CAPRIE) trial compared the efficacy of clopidogrel and aspirin in preventing ischemic events in patients with recent myocardial infarction, recent ischemic stroke, or PVD. Notably, in the 6452 patients in the PVD subgroup, clopidogrel treatment resulted in a 23.8% reduction in adverse cardiovascular events [55].

There is strong evidence to support an association between supervised exercise programs and improved blood pressure lipid and glycemic control for all patients with claudication [56]. Thus, it is a key component of a comprehensive claudication treatment program.

Cilostazol is a phosphodiesterase type 3 inhibitor and is an effective therapy to improve symptoms and increase walking distance in patients with peripheral vascular disease and intermittent claudication (in absence of heart failure). Pentoxifylline may be considered as second-line alternative therapy to cilostazol. However, the clinical effectiveness of pentoxifylline is not well established.

Endovascular interventions are indicated for individuals with lifestyle limiting disability due to intermittent claudication.

Foot ulcers

Up to 15% of diabetic patients will develop diabetic foot ulceration (Figure 6.7), of which 14–20% will require amputation. Annual treatment costs of foot care in the UK are around £13 million. Regular visual inspection and assessment of feet in diabetic patients and good education are important in preventing future foot problems. A number of risk stratification systems and care pathways have been developed and the most internationally recognized guidelines have been published by the International Working Group on the Diabetic Foot, a worldwide organization founded in 1996 [57]. The NICE guideline published in January 2004 is useful in risk stratification and provides a care pathway for the management of diabetic feet [58].

The initial assessment of diabetic foot should include detailed inspection to determine any intactness of the skin, foot deformity, abnormally shaped nails, and destructive neuroarthropathy [59]. Inspection of the skin can provide vital information about the presence of neuropathy and

Diabetic foot ulcer

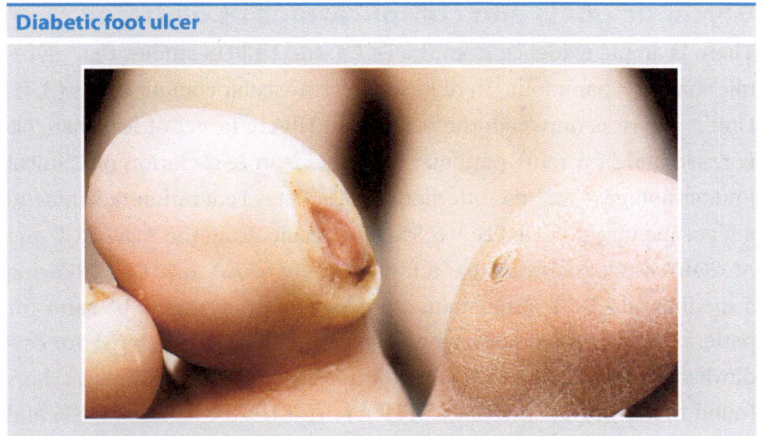

Figure 6.7 Diabetic foot ulcer. A grade 1, stage A diabetic ulcer of the right great toe. Reproduced with permission from CAPRIE Steering Committee 1996 [51].

vascular disease. Palpation of pedal pulses (both posterior tibial and dorsalis pedis) is crucial while performing risk stratification. Hand-held dopplers are increasingly being used for vascular assessment. One of the first sensory modalities to be impaired in diabetic feet is the ability to detect vibrations which has been traditionally assessed using a 128 Hz tunning fork. The use of a 10 g nylon monofilament has recently been introduced in combination of the above. Neurothesiometers, measuring vibration perception in volts, are also being used in some centers.

Patients with feet that indiciate neurovascular insufficiency are at risk for ulcers from pressure necrosis or inflammation from repeated skin stress and unnoticed minor trauma. These can evolve into cellulitis, deep tissue infections, osteomyelitis, gangrene, and may require amputation. Wounds and infected ulcers should be treated intensively with appropriate use of antibiotics, avoidance of further trauma, and revascularization where indicated to promote wound healing. Patients should be cared for by an experienced podiatrist or orthopedist.

It is often difficult to cure foot ulcers and infections and therefore prevention is extremely important. All diabetic patients should be provided information regarding foot care and should have their feet routinely risk assessed and appropriately referred to a podiatrist.

Glycemic goals and complications of diabetes

There is ample evidence from the DCCT and UKPDS studies that glycemic control is paramount in reducing microvascular complications [3,4]. Unless the risks outweigh the benefit, an HbA1c target of less than 7% is reasonable for most patients. The American Association of Clinical Endocrinologists and the International Diabetes Federation recommend a glycemic target of HbA1c <6.5%. The results from the ADVANCE and ACCORD studies suggest that a target HbA1c of 7.0 to 7.9% (achieving a median of 7.5%) rather than a median of <6.4%, may be safer for patients with long-standing type 2 diabetes who are at high risk for cardiovascular disease [44,60]. In a post-hoc analysis, ACCORD researchers found that every 1% increases in HbA1c (for HbA1c levels of 6.5% and above) was associated with a 38% higher risk of a macrovascular event, 40% higher risk of a microvascular event, and 38% higher risk of death (P <0.0001) [61].

It is necessary to aim for the lowest possible HbA1c without causing undue harm. The limiting factor is almost always hypoglycemia. A tight control should not be pursued in situations with an unfavorable risk-benefit ratio for intensive blood glucose lowering, which include advanced age, significant concomitant disease (eg, hypoglycemic unawareness, seizures, an increased risk of falling) and advanced complications.

- A continuous relationship exists between glycemia and microvascular complications, with a 35% reduction in risk for each 1% decrement in HbA1c.
- Medical practitioners should aim for the lowest possible HbA1c that does not cause undue harm to the patient.
- Vigorous blood pressure control reduces both microvascular and macrovascular events.
- The most effective approach for the prevention of macrovascular complications appears to be multifactorial risk factor reduction, encompassing glycemic control, smoking cessation, aggressive blood pressure control, and treatment of dyslipidemia.

References

1   Roglic G, Unwin N, Bennett PH. The burden of mortality attributable to diabetes: realistic estimates for the year 2000. *Diabetes Care*. 2005;28:2130-2135.

2   Diabetes Control and Complications Trial Research Group. The effect of intensive treatment of diabetes on the development and progression of long-term complications in insulin-dependent diabetes mellitus. *N Engl J Med*.1993;329:977.

3   UK Prospective Diabetes Study Group (UKPDS 33). Intensive blood glucose control with sulfonylureas or insulin compared with conventional treatment and risk of complications in patients with type 2 diabetes. *Lancet*.1998;352:837-853.

4   Setter SM, Campbell RK, Cahoon C. Biochemial pathways of microvascular complication in diabetes mellitus. *Ann Pharmacother*. 2003;37:1858-1866.

5   Kuroki T, Isshiki K, King G. Oxidative stress: the lead or supporting actor in the pathogenesis of diabetic complications. *J Am Soc Nephrol*. 2003;14:S216-220.

6   Harris MI, Klein R, Welborn TA. Onset of NIDDM occurs at least 4–7 years before clinical diagnosis. *Diabetes Care*. 1992;15:815-819.

7   Molitch ME, DeFronzo RA, Franz MJ, et al. Diabetic nephropathy. *Diabetes Care*. 2003;26:S94-8.

8   Molitch ME, DeFronzo RA, Franz MJ, et al. Nephropathy in diabetes. *Diabetes Care*. 2004;27:S79-83.

9   Mogensen CE. Microalbuminuria in prediction and prevention of diabetic nephropathy in insulin-dependent diabetes mellitus patients. *Diabetes Complics*. 1995;9:337-349.

10 Diabetes Control and Complications (DCCT) Research Group. Effect of intensive therapy on the development and progression of diabetic nephropathy in the Diabetes Control and Complications Trial. *Kidney intl*. 1995; 47:1703.

11 Bending JJ, Viberti GC, Watkins PJ, Keen H. Intermittent clinical proteinuria and renal function in diabetes: evolution and effect of glycemic control. *Br Med J*. 1986;292:83.

12 Hansen HP, Tauber-Lassen E, Jensen BR, Parving HH. Effect of dietary protein restriction on prognosis in patients with diabetic nephropathy. *Kidney Int*. 2002;6:220-228.

13 Breyer JA. Diabetic nephropathy in insulin-dependent patients. *Am J Kidney Dis*. 1992;20:533.

14 Vora JP, Ibrahim HA, Bakris GL. Responding to the challenge of diabetic nephropathy: the historic evolution of detection, prevention and management. *J Hum Hypertens*. 2000;14:667-685.

15 Adler AL, Stevens RJ, Manley SE et al. Development and progression of nephropathy in type 2 diabetes. *Kidney Intl*. 2003;63:225-232.

16 Parving HH, Hommel E. Prognosis in diabetic nephropathy. *BMJ*. 1989;299:230-233.

17 Bunce C, Wormald R. Causes of blind certifications in England and Wales April 1999 – March 2000. *Eye*. 2008;905-911.

18 Keenan HA, Costacou T, Sun JK, et al. Clinical factors associated with resistance to microvascular complications in diabetic patients of extreme disease duration: the 50-year medalist study. *Diabetes Care*. 2007;30:1995-1997.

19 Fong DS, Aiello LP, Ferris FL 3rd, Klein R. Diabetic retinopathy. *Diabetes Care*. 2004;27:2540-2553.

20 Brownlee M. Biochemistry and molecular cell biology of diabetic complications. *Nature*. 2001;414:813-820.

21 Shams N, Lanchulev T. Role of vascular endothelial growth factor in ocular angiogenesis. *Ophthalmol Clin Nth Am*. 2006;19:335-344.

22 Sunder RM, Robert H, Skyler J. *Atlas of Clinical Endocrinology*. Volume 2. London: Current Medicine Group; 1999.

23 Watkins PJ. Retinopathy. *BMJ*. 2003;326:924-926.

24 Gaede P, Vedel P, Larsen N, Jensen GV, Parving HH, Pedersen O. Multifactorial intervention and cardiovascular disease in patients with type 2 diabetes. *N Engl J Med*. 2003;348:383-393.

25 Scott R, Best J, Forder P, et al; for the FIELD Study Investigators. Fenofibrate intervention and event lowering in diabetes (FIELD) study: baseline characteristics and short-term effects of fenofibrate [ISRCTN64783481]. *Cardiovasc Diabetol*. 2005;4:13.

26 Ryan EH, Han DP, Ramsay RC. Diabetic macula edema associated with glitazone use. *Retina.* 2006;26:562-570.
27 Fong DS, Contreras R. Glitazone use associated with diabetic macular edema. *Am J Ophthalmol.* 2009;147:583-586.
28 Diabetes Control and Complications Trial Research Group. Progression of retinopathy with intensive versus conventional treatment in the Diabetes Control and Complications Trial. *Ophthalmology.* 1995;102:647.
29 Early Treatment Diabetic Retinopathy Study Research Group (ETDRS). Early photocoagulation for diabetic retinopathy. *Ophthalmology.* 1994;98:766-785.
30 Blumenkranz MD, Yellachich MS, Andersen D. New instrument: semiautomated patterned scanning laser for retinal photocoagulation. *Retina.* 2006;26:370-376.
31 Al-Hussainy S, Dodson PM, Gibson JM. Pain response and follow- up of patients undergoing panretinal laser photocoagulation with reduced exposure times. *Eye.* 2008;26:370-376.
32 Kunisaki M, Bursell SE, Clermont AC, et al. Vitamin E prevents diabetes-induced abnormal retinal blood flow via the diacylglycerol-protein kinase C pathway. *Am J Physiol.* 1995;269:e239-e246.
33 PKC-DRS2 Group. Effect of ruboxistaurin on visual loss in patients with diabetic retinopathy. *Ophthalmology.* 2006;113:2221-2230.
34 Ewing DJ. Autonomic neuropathy: its diagnosis and prognosis. *Clin Endocrinol Metab.* 1986;15:855-888.
35 Boulton A. Management of diabetic peripheral neuropathy. *Clinical Diabetes.* 2005;23:9-15.
36 Vinik A. Neuropathy: new concepts in evaluation and treatment. *South Med J.* 2002;95:21-23.
37 Duby JJ, Campbell RK. Diabetic neuropathy: an intensive review. *Am J Health-Syst Pharm.* 2004;61:160-176.
38 Wong MC, Chung JWY, Wong TKS. Effects of treatments for symptoms of painful diabetic neuropathy: systematic review. *BMJ.* 2007;335:387.
39 Grief CJ, Conn DK, Reekam RV. The treatment of chronic pain with antidepressants in older adults. *J Geriatric Care.* 2002;1:255-263.
40 Spallone V, Lacerenza M, Rossi A, Sicuteri R, Marchettini P. Painful diabetic neuropathy: approach to diagnosis and management. *Clin J Pain.* 2011; [Epub ahead of print].
41 Gimbel JS, Richards P, Portenoy RK. Controlled-release oxycodone for pain in diabetic neuropathy: A randomized controlled trial. *Neurology.* 2003;60:927-934.
42 Harati Y, Gooch C, Swenson M. Double-blind randomized trial of tramadol for the treatment of the pain of diabetic neuropathy. *Neurology.* 1998;50:1842-1846.
43 Maitra A, Abbas AK. The endocrine system. In: Kumar V, Abbas AK, Fasuto N, eds. *Pathologic Basis of Disease.* London: Elsevier; 2005:1155-1205.
44 Patel A, MacMahon S, Chalmers J, et al. Intensive blood glucose control and vascular outcomes in patients with type 2 diabetes. *N Engl J Med.* 2008;358:260-272.
45 National Institute for Health and Clinical Excellence. *Type 2 diabetes. NICE clinical guidelines 87;* 2009. www.nice.org.uk/CG87. Accessed September 5, 2012.
46 National High Blood Pressure Education Program Coordinating Committee. The Seventh Report of the Joint National Committee on Prevention, Detection, Evaluation, and Treatment of High Blood Pressure. *JAMA.* 2003;289:2560-2571.
47 Colhoun HM, Betteridge DJ, Durrington PN, et al; for the CARDS investigators. Primary prevention of cardiovascular disease with atorvastatin in type 2 diabetes in the Collaborative Atorvastatin Diabetes Study (CARDS): multicentre randomised placebo-controlled trial. *Lancet.* 2004;364:685-696.
48 Collins R, Armitage J, Heart Protection Study Collaborative Group MRC/BHF Heart Protection Study of cholesterol-lowering with simvastatin in 5963 people with diabetes: a randomised placebo-controlled trial. *Lancet.* 2003;361:2005-2016.
49 Janghorbani M, Hu FB, Willett WC, et al. Prospective study of type 1 and type 2 diabetes and risk of stroke subtypes. *Diabetes Care.* 2007;30:1730-1735.

50 Laing SP, Swerdlow AJ, Carpenter LM, et al. Mortality from cerebrovascular disease in a cohort of 23,000 patients with insulin-treated diabetes. *Stroke*. 2003;34:418-421.

51 Beckman JA, Creager MA, Libby P. Diabetes and atherosclerosis: epidemiology, pathophysiology, and management. *JAMA*. 2002;287:2570-2581.

52 Chinese Acute Stroke Trial Collaborative Group. Randomized placebo-controlled trial of early aspirin use in 20,000 patients with acute ischemic stroke. *Lancet*. 1997;349:1641.

53 Multicenter Acute Stroke Trial—Italy (MAST-I) Group. Randomized controlled trial of streptokinase, aspirin, and combination of both in treatment of acute ischemic stroke. *Lancet*. 1995;346:509.

54 Murabito JM, D'Agostino RB, Silbershatz H. Intermittent claudication. A risk profile from The Framingham Heart Study. *Circulation*. 1997;96:44-49.

55 Creager MA, Libby P. Peripheral artery disease. In: Braunwald E, Zipes DP, Libby P, eds. *Heart Disease: A Textbook of Cardiovascular Medicine*. Philadelphia: WB Saunders Company; 2001.

56 Murphy TP, Cutlip DE, Regensteiner JG, et al. Supervised exercise versus primary stenting for claudication resulting from aortoillac peripheral artery disease. *Circulation*. 2012;125:130-139.

57 International working group on the diabetic foot. *Practical and specific guidelines*. IDF website. www.iwgdf.org/index.php. Accessed September 5, 2012.

58 National Institute for Health and Clinical Excellence. *NICE clinical guideline CG10 – type 2 diabetes footcare*. www.nice.org.uk/CG10. Accessed September 5, 2012.

59 Heckman, J D, Agarwal, A, Schenck, RC. Current Orthopedic Diagnosis and Treatment. London: Springer; 1999.

60 ACCORD Study Group. Long-term effects of glucose lowering on cardiovascular outcomes. *N Engl J Med*. 2001;364:818-828.

61 Zoungas S, Chalmers J, Ninoyama T, et al. Association of HbA1c levels with vascular complications and death in patients with type 2 diabetes: evidence of glycaemic thresholds. *Diabetologia*. 2012;55:636-643.